Job's Illness:
Loss, Grief and Integration
A Psychological Interpretation

by

JACK KAHN
M.D., F.R.C.Psych., D.P.M.

with

HESTER SOLOMON, M.A.

GASKELL

© The Royal College of Psychiatrists 1986

ISBN 0 902241 17 6

Gaskell is an imprint of the Royal College of
Psychiatrists, 17 Belgrave Square, London SW1

First published 1975 by Pergamon Press Ltd
Reprinted 1986

Printed in Britain at the Alden Press, Oxford

Contents

"Solomon and Job have known best and
spoken best of man's misery; the one
most fortunate, the other the most
unfortunate of men; the one knowing
by experience the emptiness of
pleasure; the other the reality of sorrow."

    PASCAL'S *Pensees*, No. 357

"I have been young, and now am not too old,
And I have seen the righteous forsaken,
His health, his honour and his quality taken.
This is not what we were formerly told."

    EDMUND BLUNDEN

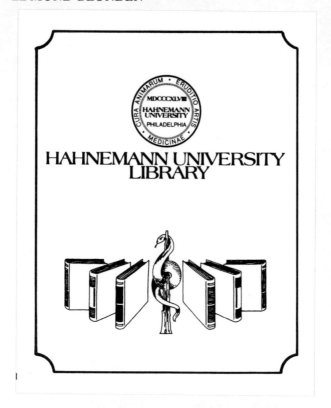

Preface

The re-issue of this book by the Royal College of Psychiatrists under the Gaskell imprint is a source of pleasure and pride to me. At the time of its publication, in 1975, I was about to retire from the clinical post which I had held in the London Borough of Newham. I had no foreknowledge of the various post-retirement assignments that subsequently came to me. This book opened a new chapter in my life.

I began to receive letters from friends and strangers, who were glad to reveal thoughts about the Book of Job which they had kept private over the years, as if waiting to share them with someone who had shown similar interest.

Many correspondents referred to interpretations relating to personal experiences. One introduced me to *Blake's Vision of the Book of Job* by Joseph Wickstead[1] (now sadly out of print), which gives a detailed analysis of Blake's engravings.

I had previously become acquainted with Blake's engravings through the work of Marion Milner. Wickstead's book gave me a stimulus to immerse myself in the works of Blake. How reassuring it became, at the age of 70 + , to find something new to study and enjoy!

I had concluded the original introduction with the thought that

"Even after depositing the manuscript with the publishers, new ideas came to notice and new comparisons came to the mind. My hope now is that readers will be able to take over some of the pleasure of the discovery of new growing points."

This hope was amply fulfilled. I had suggested that the prologue, in which God challenges Satan over the perfection of Job, took place in the mind of Job. How else could such a virtuous person have been permitted to undergo such sufferings?

One correspondent carried this idea a considerable stage further. She suggested that the death of Job's children, too, was in the mind of Job, and that that is why, in the epilogue, a new family could so miraculously appear. She, herself, had had a comparable experience. At the age of 41 she had suffered a severe depressive illness and, during its most severe stage, she imagined that her children were dead. On her recovery, she says "I saw my daughters with new delight.

[1]Joseph H. Wickstead, *Blake's Vision of the Book of Job* (London: J. M. Dent and Sons Limited, 1910).

vii

There were never such beautiful children". She added "Could Job's particular emphasis on the daughters be because he had least valued them before?"

I have continued to be preoccupied with the contribution of the comforters which, in my view, has been consistently undervalued by Bible commentators. Comparisons can be made between the rounds of speeches with Job and ideas of group therapy. Their words were a reflection of Job's own former views in his original state of perfection. Together, they subscribed to the ideas of moral determinism, in which the good life deserves the good reward, and bad fortune is the proof of a bad character. This was the point at which Job parted company with what he had been formerly told, because he held fast to his integrity.

Determinism is an important stage in the study of the development of the human condition and its environment. Moral determinism came first, and was succeeded by physical determinism, in which the same causes always lead to the same effects; and this gives a foundation for scientific studies and the "laws" which are discovered. Next came psychological determinism, as promulgated by Freud. It requires a further conceptual leap to go beyond determinism and to allow for chance.

Here I wish to refer to Elihu, who made his contribution after the comforters were eventually silenced by Job. The passages relating to Elihu are considered by modern Bible commentators to be a later and irrelevant interpolation into the text. Moses Maimonides, on the other hand, attached fundamental importance to Elihu's views. To me, his contribution appears to be the one which allows Job to escape from determinism.

The rapid recent increase of knowledge leads many people to believe that whatever is at present unknown will, in time, be revealed; that events are unpredictable only to the extent that we have not yet acquired sufficient knowledge, but that this in time will come. This does not take into account the fact that there are themes in which unpredictability is the very essence. The lesson of Job is that he originally believed that his perfection could control his fate, and guarantee good fortune. This is the moral determinism which should enable Man to control God and, in its scientific equivalent, is the hubris of the search for absolute certainty.

Job's recovery was an inner consummation which came when the Lord answered Job out of the whirlwind (N. E. V. Tempest). The recovery was a reconciliation of opposites: of love and hate; of goodness and badness; of virtue and sin; of illness and health. Similarly, Prospero's island exile began with a tempest and ended with a tempest, and the consummation was Prospero's abrogation of his omnipotence.

Job's final position was attained by access to shame and awe:

> "Therefore I melt away
> I repent in dust and ashes"
> (N.E.V.)

The awe was Job's tribute to destiny, which helps people to accommodate to events which they cannot control, and is the final acknowledgement of the mortality of Man.

Introduction

WHEN an idea has occupied the mind for some twenty-five years it is quite a wrench to part with it and present it publicly in the form of a book. And yet the thoughts must be put at risk if they are to be allowed to have a life of their own.

At one level this book represents my experience of psychiatry—beginning with my entry into the profession and extending to the point when its acceptance for publication coincided with my retirement from my post in the London Borough of Newham.

At a somewhat deeper level, the book represents the converging of the Hebrew heritage which came in my childhood through my father (who seems to have taught me more than I remember having learned), with the general literary and scientific environment to which I was exposed in my adult life.

The ideas in this book began to take shape in 1948. Only a short time before this I had taken the step of leaving general practice and I was receiving a training in psychiatry. The most immediate stimulus to my rereading of the Book of Job came from the account given to me by a patient assigned to me for psychotherapy. As his story unfolded, detail after detail, it brought recollections to me of the Book of Job. I had recently acquired the Soncino Version, published in England in 1946, and containing the Hebrew text, an English translation, and a commentary drawn together from a variety of Jewish and Christian sources. I did not actually turn to the text until the interval between written and oral examination in psychiatry. The linkages of ideas were made stronger by the fact that in the examination I had had to write an essay on "The Integration of the Personality", and perhaps it was associations with ideas worked out under stress that led to the thought that Job's initial "perfection" was intended to convey the same quality as is implied by the word "integration".

In 1953 I ventured to give, but not to publish, my first paper on the subject. It was presented to a group of colleagues who shared the intensity of my interest to such an extent that the discussion had to be continued at the next meeting. I had, however, no wish to enclose the ideas in a form that would seem suitable for publication. It was as if I wished to avoid finality in something which was still finding a shape in my thoughts.

Gradually I became aware of the wealth of references to the Book of Job in general literature, and many of them were discovered by chance while browsing in bookshops, rather than by deliberate search. It was chance that took me to a performance of *J.B.* by Archibald MacLeish, on a visit to the Exposition Universelle Internationale in Brussels in 1958. It was being presented by the Yale University School of Drama in the American Pavilion. The programme notes which I preserved include:

> Man, the scientists say, is the animal that thinks. They are wrong. Man is the animal that loves. It is in man's love that God exists and triumphs: in man's love that life is beautiful: in man's love that the world's injustice is resolved. To hold together in one thought those terrible opposites of good and evil which struggle in the world is to be capable of life, and only love will hold them so.
>
> Our labor always, like Job's labor, is to learn through suffering to love . . . to love even that which let us suffer.

Five years later, on a visit to the United States of America, it was by chance again that I found the published text of the play.

On several occasions it occurred to me to organize my ideas on the subject, and use the Book of Job as an illustration of basic human problems which patients describe when being treated for psychiatric disorders. I continued to be impressed by the frequency with which the words that patients used resembled those of Job. It also became apparent that the expression of these ideas was an indication of some change in the patient's mental state—often for the better. What was being conveyed was a search for a new level of integration which, when achieved, seemed to be an improvement on the previous balance of mind which had been upset. Job himself seemed to represent the efforts of many present-day sufferers to reach levels of maturity which were as yet unattained.

If I had written the book at the time when it was first contemplated, it would not have included the accretions which may either obscure or add further illustrations to the original ideas.

The undertaking took longer than expected. The first few chapters came comparatively easily from somewhat frequently repeated associations of ideas. Later chapters formed themselves more slowly, and ideas changed at the point of the pen or, more accurately, at the moment of dictation. At this stage I was fortunate in engaging the services of Mrs. Hester Solomon (a graduate in literature and philosophy) for secretarial and editorial assistance. She was captured by the language and the magical mysteries of the Bible text. As time went on, dictation became discussion of the ideas which were entering the script. She added to the ideas and it is with gratitude to her that I acknowledge her assistance on the title page.

The time had come to go beyond chance, and to hew out meaning, verse by verse, from the Bible text. Different Bible versions were compared. Different commentaries were consulted.

There still remained the fortunate chance element in the possession of many relevant books from my father's library and from some rather haphazard collecting of my own. Recollections came, during the course of writing, from books which I had read some thirty or forty years previously. One of the most recent purchases was the Septuagint Bible in the translation of Charles Thompson, which gave one or two unexpected glimpses into Job's background. It was there that I found the reference to "children of my concubines". It was there, also, that I found confirmation of a rather over-stretched interpretation of my own which I gave to some words of MacLeish's *J.B.* Sarah asks: "Has death no meaning? Pain no meaning?", and this took my thoughts to the labour pains which should have given Job's wife a claim to a grief which the Authorized Version does not record. The Septuagint Version, however, speaks directly of "those sons and daughters, whom I brought forth with pangs and sorrow, and for whom I toiled in vain . . .".

The New English Bible Version was chosen for the verse-by-verse account of Job's progress, and I am grateful to its publishers for permission to reprint it here. The reader will be able to turn from the propositions in this book back to the context from which they were derived. At the same time, the words of the Authorized Version will no doubt reverberate in the reader's mind as an accompaniment to any other text. There is something special about the Authorized Version. Its phrases have passed into the language of the people and have shaped the idioms of ordinary speech. Its metaphors live on in the spoken word, even of those who have no knowledge of the source. This is not the result of deliberate choice, but rather that, at the time that the Authorized Version was published, the general population derived its formal language from regular readings in religious services.

The consequence is that the Authorized Version has provided some general characteristics of the English language, and has contributed to the shaping of the vocabulary in which individual thoughts are expressed. The corollary is that some Bible phrases are used in a totality in which the meaning of the individual words is lost. The use of the New English Version compels us to give fresh thought to what the words mean. It provides unexpected clarification of many obscure passages and even though, in places, one misses the majesty of the Authorized Version, the comparison of the two versions is most rewarding.

It was in the New English Version that the Lord answered Job out of the "tempest", and not the "whirlwind". But it was in the Authorized Version that, at the beginning of Job's illness, the "tempest" bore down upon him (New English Version: "for he bears hard on me").

The work continued. Comparisons were made verse by verse, and in this endeavour Mrs. Solomon made creative and constructive contributions. At times we seemed to struggle together along with Job's struggle, sometimes arriving at an impasse in which it was possible to savour Job's depression. Eventually we came to feel that we had entered into the skin of Job and had endured the turmoil of the tempest.

Comparisons of the writings of different schools of psychiatry proved as rewarding as the comparison of different versions of the Bible. The descriptions by traditional psychiatrists of the symptoms of mental disorder paraphrased at times Job's account of his sufferings (symptoms). The psychodynamics of Freud, Melanie Klein, Winnicott and Marion Milner were drawn upon for ideas on Job's experience of grief.

In yet another dimension, the reciprocal relationship of Job and his comforters could be related to the contentions of those who look upon mental disorder as a label conveniently attached to those whose behaviour is disapproved of by representatives of the prevailing culture.

It has been a personal aim of mine to find connecting threads in the different schools of psychology and psychiatry. Descriptions in the Bible text transcend the boundaries of the different schools, and our interpretations can take the reader into a number of dimensions of present-day psychiatric theory.

At one time, a psychiatric interpretation of Job's illness would have been expected to lead to a diagnosis of a specific psychiatric illness. Even today, many psychiatrists would maintain that differential diagnosis is the most important practical preliminary to treatment. For them, each specific disease is separate from normality and separate from other diseases. My view, expressed elsewhere,[1] is that there is another approach to psychiatry in which value is attached to finding similarities in the different psychiatric syndromes. It is also possible to trace within each normal individual something of any experience which is characteristic of different psychotic conditions. The story of Job helps us to discover the links between obsessional states, depression, and paranoia; and it also allows us to consider the personal variations which exist, in each culture, on the borderland of sanity. Thus, it is possible to find some support for those writers who challenge the reality behind psychiatric labels, but one does not have to follow these writers in abandoning the search for external standards by which to judge the perversities of inner experiences. A mental disorder can be a creative experience and it was through suffering that Job achieved his new level of integration. But for many people the suffering which is involved in mental disorder is too high a price for anything that is achieved.

It would be a misreading of the lesson of Job to leave it entirely in a psychiatric dimension, and it would be illusory to think of loss and grief as being invariably a prelude to successful integration. Psychiatric interpretation and treatment cannot demand success; and there are literary, philosophical, and religious interpretations of human problems in which success is not the final aim. Job is Everyman and every man is Job. Job's experience of himself is an introduction to every enquiry into the meaning of existence.

The most difficult task was to bring the book to a conclusion. Even after depositing the manuscript with the publishers, new ideas came to notice and new comparisons came to the mind.

My hope now is that readers will be able to take over some of the pleasure of the discovery of new growing points.

J. H. KAHN

[1] J. H. Kahn, "Dimensions of diagnosis and treatment", *Mental Hygiene*, **53** (2) (1969), pp. 229–236.

THE BOOK OF
JOB

Prologue

1 THERE LIVED IN THE LAND OF UZ a man of blameless
and upright life named Job, who feared God and set his face against
2 3 wrongdoing. He had seven sons and three daughters; and he owned
seven thousand sheep and three thousand camels, five hundred yoke of
oxen and five hundred asses, with a large number of slaves. Thus Job was
the greatest man in all the East.

4 Now his sons used to foregather and give, each in turn, a feast in his
own house; and they used to send and invite their three sisters to eat and
5 drink with them. Then, when a round of feasts was finished, Job sent for
his children and sanctified them, rising early in the morning and sacrificing
a whole-offering for each of them; for he thought that they might somehow
have sinned against God and committed blasphemy in their hearts. This
he always did.

6 The day came when the members of the court of heaven took their
places in the presence of the LORD, and Satan*a* was there among them.
7 The LORD asked him where he had been. 'Ranging over the earth', he said,
8 'from end to end.' Then the LORD asked Satan, 'Have you considered my
servant Job? You will find no one like him on earth, a man of blameless
and upright life, who fears God and sets his face against wrongdoing.'
9 Satan answered the LORD, 'Has not Job good reason to be God-fearing?
10 Have you not hedged him round on every side with your protection,
him and his family and all his possessions? Whatever he does you have
11 blessed, and his herds have increased beyond measure. But stretch out your
hand and touch all that he has, and then he will curse you to your face.'
12 Then the LORD said to Satan, 'So be it. All that he has is in your hands;
only Job himself you must not touch.' And Satan left the LORD's presence.
13 When the day came that Job's sons and daughters were eating and drink-
14 ing in the eldest brother's house, a messenger came running to Job and
15 said, 'The oxen were ploughing and the asses were grazing near them, when
the Sabaeans swooped down and carried them off, after putting the herds-
16 men to the sword; and I am the only one to escape and tell the tale.' While
he was still speaking, another messenger arrived and said, 'God's fire
flashed from heaven. It struck the sheep and the shepherds and burnt them
17 up; and I am the only one to escape and tell the tale.' While he was still
speaking, another arrived and said, 'The Chaldaeans, three bands of them,
have made a raid on the camels and carried them off, after putting the drivers

a Or the adversary.

to the sword; and I am the only one to escape and tell the tale.' While this 18
man was speaking, yet another arrived and said, 'Your sons and daughters
were eating and drinking in the eldest brother's house, when suddenly a 19
whirlwind swept across from the desert and struck the four corners of the
house, and it fell on the young people and killed them; and I am the only
one to escape and tell the tale.' At this Job stood up and rent his cloak; then 20
he shaved his head and fell prostrate on the ground, saying: 21

> Naked I came from the womb,
> naked I shall return whence I came.
> The LORD gives and the LORD takes away;
> blessed be the name of the LORD.

Throughout all this Job did not sin; he did not charge God with unreason. 22
  Once again the day came when the members of the court of heaven took 2
their places in the presence of the LORD, and Satan was there among them.
The LORD asked him where he had been. 'Ranging over the earth', he said, 2
'from end to end.' Then the LORD asked Satan, 'Have you considered my 3
servant Job? You will find no one like him on earth, a man of blameless and
upright life, who fears God and sets his face against wrongdoing. You
incited me to ruin him without a cause, but his integrity is still unshaken.'
Satan answered the LORD, 'Skin for skin! There is nothing the man will 4
grudge to save himself. But stretch out your hand and touch his bone and 5
his flesh, and see if he will not curse you to your face.'
  Then the LORD said to Satan, 'So be it. He is in your hands; but spare 6
his life.' And Satan left the LORD's presence, and he smote Job with running 7
sores from head to foot, so that he took a piece of a broken pot to scratch 8
himself as he sat among the ashes. Then his wife said to him, 'Are you still 9
unshaken in your integrity? Curse God and die!' But he answered, 'You 10
talk as any wicked fool of a woman might talk. If we accept good from God,
shall we not accept evil?' Throughout all this, Job did not utter one sinful
word.
  When Job's three friends, Eliphaz of Teman, Bildad of Shuah, and 11
Zophar of Naamah, heard of all these calamities which had overtaken him,
they left their homes and arranged to come and condole with him and
comfort him. But when they first saw him from a distance, they did not 12
recognize him; and they wept aloud, rent their cloaks and tossed dust into
the air over their heads. For seven days and seven nights they sat beside 13
him on the ground, and none of them said a word to him; for they saw that
his suffering was very great.

Job's complaint to God

After this Job broke silence and cursed the day of his birth: 3 1-2

> Perish the day when I was born   3
> and the night which said, 'A man is conceived'!
> May that day turn to darkness; may God above not look for it,   4
> nor light of dawn shine on it.

5   May blackness sully it, and murk and gloom,
    cloud smother that day, swift darkness eclipse its sun.
6   Blind darkness swallow up that night;
    count it not among the days of the year,
    reckon it not in the cycle of the months.
7   That night, may it be barren for ever,
    no cry of joy be heard in it.
8   Cursed be it by those whose magic binds even the monster of the deep,
    who are ready to tame Leviathan himself with spells.
9   May no star shine out in its twilight;
    may it wait for a dawn that never comes,
    nor ever see the eyelids of the morning,
10 because it did not shut the doors of the womb that bore me
    and keep trouble away from my sight.
11 Why was I not still-born,
    why did I not die when I came out of the womb?
12 Why was I ever laid on my mother's knees
    or put to suck at her breasts?
16 Why was I not hidden like an untimely birth,
    like an infant that has not lived to see the light?
13 For then I should be lying in the quiet grave,
    asleep in death, at rest,
14 with kings and their ministers
    who built themselves palaces,
15 with princes rich in gold
    who filled their houses with silver.
17*a* There the wicked man chafes no more,
    there the tired labourer rests;
18 the captive too finds peace there
    and hears no taskmaster's voice;
19 high and low are there,
    even the slave, free from his master.

20 Why should the sufferer be born to see the light?
    Why is life given to men who find it so bitter?
21 They wait for death but it does not come,
    they seek it more eagerly than *b* hidden treasure.
22 They are glad when they reach the tomb,
    and when they come to the grave they exult.
23 Why should a man be born to wander blindly,
    hedged in by God on every side?
24 My sighing is all my food,
    and groans pour from me in a torrent.
25 Every terror that haunted me has caught up with me,
    and all that I feared has come upon me.
26 There is no peace of mind nor quiet for me;
    I chafe in torment and have no rest.

a Verse 16 transposed to follow verse 12.   *b Or seek it among . . .*

First cycle of speeches

Then Eliphaz the Temanite began: 4

If one ventures to speak with you, will you lose patience? 2
For who could hold his tongue any longer?
Think how once you encouraged those who faltered, 3
how you braced feeble arms,
how a word from you upheld the stumblers 4
and put strength into weak knees.
But now that adversity comes upon you, you lose patience; 5
it touches you, and you are unmanned.
Is your religion no comfort to you? 6
Does your blameless life give you no hope?
For consider, what innocent man has ever perished? 7
Where have you seen the upright destroyed?
This I know, that those who plough mischief and sow trouble 8
reap as they have sown;
they perish at the blast of God 9
and are shrivelled by the breath of his nostrils.

The roar of the lion, the whimpering of his cubs, fall silent; 10
the teeth of the young lions are broken;
the lion perishes for lack of prey 11
and the whelps of the lioness are abandoned.

A word stole into my ears, 12
and they caught the whisper of it;
in the anxious visions of the night, 13
when a man sinks into deepest sleep,
terror seized me and shuddering; 14
the trembling of my body frightened me.
A wind brushed my face 15
and made the hairs bristle on my flesh;
and a figure stood there whose shape I could not discern, 16
an apparition loomed before me,
and I heard the sound of a low voice:
'Can mortal man be more righteous than God, 17
or the creature purer than his Maker?
If God mistrusts his own servants 18
and finds his messengers at fault,
how much more those that dwell in houses whose walls are clay, 19
whose foundations are dust,
which can be crushed like a bird's nest
or torn down between dawn and dark, 20
how much more shall such men perish outright and unheeded,
a die, without ever finding wisdom?' 21

a Prob. rdg.; transposing Their rich possessions are snatched from them *to follow 5. 4.*

5   Call if you will; is there any to answer you?
    To which of the holy ones will you turn?
2   The fool is destroyed by his own angry passions,
    and the end of childish resentment is death.
3   I have seen it for myself: a fool uprooted,
    his home in sudden ruin about him,*a*
4   his children past help,
    browbeaten in court with none to save them.
5   *b* Their rich possessions are snatched from them;
    what they have harvested others hungrily devour;
    the stronger man seizes it from the panniers,
    panting, thirsting for their wealth.
6   Mischief does not grow out of the soil
    nor trouble spring from the earth;
7   man is born to trouble,
    as surely as birds fly*c* upwards.

8   For my part, I would make my petition to God
    and lay my cause before him,
9   who does great and unsearchable things,
    marvels without number.
10 He gives rain to the earth
    and sends water on the fields;
11 he raises the lowly to the heights,
    the mourners are uplifted by victory;
12 he frustrates the plots of the crafty,
    and they win no success,
13 he traps the cunning in their craftiness,
    and the schemers' plans are thrown into confusion.
14 In the daylight they run into darkness,
    and grope at midday as though it were night.
15 He saves the destitute from their greed,
    and the needy from the grip of the strong;
16 so the poor hope again,
    and the unjust are sickened.

17 Happy the man whom God rebukes!
    therefore do not reject the discipline of the Almighty.
18 For, though he wounds, he will bind up;
    the hands that smite will heal.
19 You may meet disaster six times, and he will save you;
    seven times, and no harm shall touch you.
20 In time of famine he will save you from death,
    in battle from the sword.
21 You will be shielded from the lash of slander,*d*
    and when violence comes you need not fear.

a ruin about him: *prob. rdg.; Heb. obscure.*   *b* *Line transposed from 4. 21.*
c *Or as sparks shoot.*   *d* from ... slander: *or when slander is rife.*

You will laugh at violence and starvation 22
and have no need to fear wild beasts;
for you have a covenant with the stones to spare your fields, 23
and the weeds have been constrained to leave you at peace.
You will know that all is well with your household, 24
you will look round your home and find nothing amiss;
you will know, too, that your descendants will be many 25
and your offspring like grass, thick upon the earth.
You will come in sturdy old age to the grave 26
as sheaves come in due season to the threshing-floor.

We have inquired into all this, and so it is; 27
this we have heard, and you may know it for the truth.

Then Job answered: **6**

O that the grounds for my resentment might be weighed, 2
and my misfortunes set with them on the scales!
For they would outweigh the sands of the sea: 3
what wonder if my words are wild? *a*
The arrows of the Almighty find their mark in me, 4
and their poison soaks into my spirit;
God's onslaughts wear me away.
Does the wild ass bray when he has grass 5
or the ox low when he has fodder?
Can a man eat tasteless food unseasoned with salt, 6
or find any flavour in the juice of mallows?
Food that should nourish me sticks in my throat, 7
and my bowels rumble with an echoing sound.

O that I might have my request, 8
that God would grant what I hope for:
that he would be pleased to crush me, 9
to snatch me away with his hand and cut me off!
For that would bring me relief, 10
and in the face of unsparing anguish I would leap for joy. *b*
Have I the strength to wait? 11
What end have I to expect, that I should be patient?
Is my strength the strength of stone, 12
or is my flesh bronze?
Oh how shall I find help within myself? 13
The power to aid myself is put out of my reach.

Devotion is due from his friends 14
to one who despairs and loses faith in the Almighty;
but my brothers have been treacherous as a mountain stream, 15
like the channels of streams that run dry,

a what . . . wild?: *or therefore words fail me.*   *b Prob. rdg.; Heb. adds* I have not
denied the words of the Holy One.

16   which turn dark with ice
        or are hidden with piled-up snow;
17   or they vanish the moment they are in spate,
        dwindle in the heat and are gone.
18   Then the caravans, winding hither and thither,
        go up into the wilderness and perish;[a]
19   the caravans of Tema look for their waters,
        travelling merchants of Sheba hope for them;
20   but they are disappointed, for all their confidence,
        they reach them only to be balked.
21   So treacherous have you now been to me:[b]
        you felt dismay and were afraid.
22   Did I ever say, 'Give me this or that;
        open your purses to save my life;
23   rescue me from my enemy;
        ransom me out of the hands of ruthless men'?

24   Tell me plainly, and I will listen in silence;
        show me where I have erred.
25   How harsh are the words of the upright man!
        What do the arguments of wise men[c] prove?
26   Do you mean to argue about words
        or to sift the utterance of a man past hope?
27   Would you assail an orphan[d]?
        Would you hurl yourselves on a friend?
28   So now, I beg you, turn and look at me:
        am I likely to lie to your faces?
29   Think again, let me have no more injustice;
        think again, for my integrity is in question.
30   Do I ever give voice to injustice?
        Does my sense not warn me when my words are wild?

7   Has not man hard service on earth,
        and are not his days like those of a hired labourer,
2   like those of a slave longing for the shade
        or a servant kept waiting for his wages?
3   So months of futility are my portion,
        troubled nights are my lot.
4   When I lie down, I think,
        'When will it be day that I may rise?'
        When the evening grows long and I lie down,
        I do nothing but toss till morning twilight.
5   My body is infested with worms,
        and scabs cover my skin.[e]
6   My days are swifter than a shuttle [f]
        and come to an end as the thread runs out. [g]

---

[a] *Or* and are lost.   [b] So . . . to me: *prob. rdg.; Heb. obscure.*   [c] wise men: *prob. rdg.; Heb. unintelligible.*   [d] *Or* a blameless man.   [e] *Prob. rdg.; Heb. adds* it is cracked and discharging.   [f] *Or* a fleeting odour.   [g] as . . . out: *or* without hope.

Remember, my life is but a breath of wind; 7
I shall never again see good days.
Thou wilt behold me no more with a seeing eye; 8
under thy very eyes I shall disappear.
As clouds break up and disperse, 9
so he that goes down to Sheol never comes back;
he never returns home again, 10
and his place will know him no more.*a*

But I will not hold my peace; 11
I will speak out in the distress of my mind
and complain in the bitterness of my soul.
Am I the monster of the deep, am I the sea-serpent, 12
that thou settest a watch over me?
When I think that my bed will comfort me, 13
that sleep will relieve my complaining,
thou dost terrify me with dreams 14
and affright me with visions.
I would rather be choked outright; 15
I would prefer death to all my sufferings.
I am in despair, I would not go on living; 16
leave me alone, for my life is but a vapour.
What is man that thou makest much of him 17
and turnest thy thoughts towards him,
only to punish him morning by morning 18
or to test him every hour of the day?
Wilt thou not look away from me for an instant? 19
Wilt thou not let me be while I swallow my spittle?
If I have sinned, how do I injure thee, 20
thou watcher of the hearts of men?
Why hast thou made me thy butt,
and why have I become thy target?
Why dost thou not pardon my offence 21
and take away my guilt?
But now I shall lie down in the grave;
seek me, and I shall not be.

Then Bildad the Shuhite began: **8**

How long will you say such things, 2
the long-winded ramblings of an old man?
Does God pervert judgement? 3
Does the Almighty pervert justice?
Your sons sinned against him, 4
so he left them to be victims of their own iniquity.
If only you will seek God betimes 5
and plead for the favour of the Almighty,

a Or and he will not be noticed any more in his place.

6   if you are innocent and upright,
     then indeed will he watch over you
     and see your just intent fulfilled.

7   Then, though your beginnings were humble,
     your end will be great.

8   Inquire now of older generations
     and consider the experience of their fathers;

9   for we ourselves are of yesterday and are transient;
     our days on earth are a shadow.

10   Will not they speak to you and teach you
     and pour out the wisdom of their hearts?

11   Can rushes grow where there is no marsh?
     Can reeds flourish without water?

12   While they are still in flower and not ready to cut, *a*
     they wither earlier than *b* any green plant.

13   Such is the fate of all who forget God;
     the godless man's life-thread breaks off;

14   his confidence is gossamer,
     and the ground of his trust a spider's web.

15   He leans against his house but it does not stand;
     he clutches at it but it does not hold firm.

16   His is the lush growth of a plant in the sun,
     pushing out shoots over the garden;

17   but its roots become entangled in a stony patch
     and run against a bed of rock.

18   Then someone uproots it from its place,
     which *c* disowns it and says, 'I have never known you.'

19   That is how its life withers away,
     and other plants spring up from the earth.

20   Be sure, God will not spurn the blameless man,
     nor will he grasp the hand of the wrongdoer.

21   He will yet fill your mouth with laughter,
     and shouts of joy will be on your lips;

22   your enemies shall be wrapped in confusion,
     and the tents of the wicked shall vanish away.

9   Then Job answered:

2   Indeed this I know for the truth,
     that no man can win his case against God.

3   If a man chooses to argue with him,
     God will not answer one question in a thousand. *d*

4   He is wise, he is powerful;
     what man has stubbornly resisted him and survived?

---

a and . . . cut: *or* they are surely cut.   *b Or* wither like . . .   *c Or* and.
d If a man . . . thousand: *or* If God is pleased to argue with him, man cannot answer one question in a thousand.

It is God who moves mountains, giving them no rest,   5
turning them over in his wrath;
who makes the earth start from its place   6
so that its pillars are convulsed;
who commands the sun's orb not to rise   7
and shuts up the stars under his seal;
who by himself spread out the heavens   8
and trod on the sea-monster's back; *a*
who made Aldebaran and Orion,   9
the Pleiades and the circle of the southern stars;
who does great and unsearchable things,   10
marvels without number.

He passes by me, and I do not see him;   11
he moves on his way undiscerned by me;
if he hurries on, who can bring him back?   12
Who will ask him what he does?
God does not turn back his wrath;   13
the partisans of Rahab lie prostrate at his feet.
How much less can I answer him   14
or find words to dispute with him?
Though I am right, I get no answer,   15
though I plead with my accuser for mercy.
If I summoned him to court and he responded,   16
I do not believe that he would listen to my plea—
for he bears hard upon me for a trifle   17
and rains blows on me without cause;
he leaves me no respite to recover my breath   18
but fills me with bitter thoughts.
If the appeal is to force, see how strong he is;   19
if to justice, who can compel him to give me a hearing?
Though I am right, he condemns me out of my own mouth;   20
though I am blameless, he twists my words.
Blameless, I say; of myself   21
I reck nothing, I hold my life cheap.
But it is all one; therefore I say,   22
'He destroys blameless and wicked alike.'
When a sudden flood brings death,   23
he mocks the plight of the innocent.
The land is given over to the power of the wicked,   24
and the eyes of its judges are blindfold. *b*

My days have been swifter than a runner,   25
they have slipped away and seen no prosperity;
they have raced by like reed-built skiffs,   26
swift as vultures swooping on carrion.

---

a *Or on the crests of the waves.*   *b* *Prob. rdg.; Heb. adds* if not he, then who?

27 If I think, 'I will forget my griefs,
   I will show a cheerful face and smile',
28 I tremble in every nerve;[a]
   I know that thou wilt not hold me innocent.
29 If I am to be accounted guilty,
   why do I labour in vain?
30 Though I wash myself with soap
   or cleanse my hands with lye,
31 thou wilt thrust me into the mud
   and my clothes will make me loathsome.

32 He is not a man as I am, that I can answer him
   or that we can confront one another in court.
33 If only there were one to arbitrate between us
   and impose his authority on us both,
34 so that God might take his rod from my back,
   and terror of him might not come on me suddenly.
35 I would then speak without fear of him;
   for I know I am not what I am thought to be.

10 I am sickened of life;
   I will give free rein to my griefs,
   I will speak out in bitterness of soul.
2 I will say to God, 'Do not condemn me,
   but tell me the ground of thy complaint against me.
3 Dost thou find any advantage in oppression,
   in spurning the fruit of all thy labour
   and smiling on the policy of wicked men?
4 Hast thou eyes of flesh
   or dost thou see as mortal man sees?
5 Are thy days as those of a mortal
   or thy years as the life of a man,
6 that thou lookest for guilt in me
   and dost seek in me for sin,
7 though thou knowest that I am guiltless
   and have none to save me from thee?

8 'Thy hands gave me shape and made me;
   and dost thou at once turn and destroy me?
9 Remember that thou didst knead me like clay;
   and wouldst thou turn me back into dust?
10 Didst thou not pour me out like milk
   and curdle me like cheese,
11 clothe me with skin and flesh
   and knit me together with bones and sinews?
12 Thou hast given me life and continuing favour,
   and thy providence has watched over my spirit.

[a] *Or* I am afraid of all that I must suffer.

Yet this was the secret purpose of thy heart,   13
and I know that this was thy intent:
that, if I sinned, thou wouldst be watching me   14
and wouldst not acquit me of my guilt.
If I indeed am wicked, the worse for me!   15
If I am righteous, even so I may lift up my head; *a*
if I am proud as a lion, thou dost hunt me down   16
and dost confront me again with marvellous power;
thou dost renew thy onslaught upon me,   17
and with mounting anger against me
bringest fresh forces to the attack.
Why didst thou bring me out of the womb?   18
O that I had ended there and no eye had seen me,
that I had been carried from the womb to the grave   19
and were as though I had not been born.
Is not my life short and fleeting?   20
Let me be, that I may be happy for a moment,
before I depart to a land of gloom,   21
a land of deep darkness, never to return,
a land of gathering shadows, of deepening darkness,   22
lit by no ray of light, *b* dark *c* upon dark.'

Then Zophar the Naamathite began: **11**

Should this spate of words not be answered?   2
Must a man of ready tongue be always right?
Is your endless talk to reduce men to silence?   3
Are you to talk nonsense and no one rebuke you?
You claim that your opinions are sound;   4
you say to God, 'I am spotless in thy sight.'
But if only he would speak   5
and open his lips to talk with you,
and expound to you the secrets of wisdom,   6
for wonderful are its effects!
[Know then that God exacts from you less than your sin deserves.]
Can you fathom the mystery of God,   7
can you fathom the perfection of the Almighty?
It is higher than heaven; you can do nothing.   8
It is deeper than Sheol; you can know nothing.
Its measure is longer than the earth   9
and broader than the sea.
If he passes by, he may keep secret his passing;   10
if he proclaims it, who can turn him back?
He surely knows which men are false,   11
and when he sees iniquity, does he not take note of it? *d*

---

a Prob. rdg.; Heb. adds filled with shame and steeped in my affliction.   *b* lit . . .
light: *or* a place of disorder.   *c Prob. rdg.; Heb. obscure.*   *d* does . . . of it?:
or he does not stand aloof.

12   Can a fool grow wise?
        can a wild ass's foal be born a man?

13   If only you had directed your heart rightly
        and spread out your hands to pray to him!

14   If you have wrongdoing in hand, thrust it away;
        let no iniquity make its home with you.

15   Then you could hold up your head without fault,
        a man of iron, knowing no fear.

16   Then you will forget your trouble;
        you will remember it only as flood-waters that have passed;

17   life will be lasting, bright as noonday,
        and darkness will be turned to morning.

18   You will be confident, because there is hope;
        sure of protection, you will lie down in confidence;[a]

19   great men will seek your favour.

20   Blindness will fall on the wicked;
        the ways of escape are closed to them,
        and their hope is despair.

12 Then Job answered:

2   No doubt you are perfect men[b]
        and absolute wisdom is yours!

3   But I have sense as well as you;
        in nothing do I fall short of you;
        what gifts indeed have you that others have not?

4   Yet I am a laughing-stock to my friend—
        a laughing-stock, though I am innocent and blameless,
        one that called upon God, and he answered.[c]

5   Prosperity and ease look down on misfortune,
        on the blow that fells the man who is already reeling,

6   while the marauders' tents are left undisturbed
        and those who provoke God live safe and sound. [d]

7   Go and ask the cattle,
        ask the birds of the air to inform you,

8   or tell the creatures that crawl to teach you,
        and the fishes of the sea to give you instruction.

9   Who cannot learn from all these
        that the LORD's own hand has done this?

11[e] (Does not the ear test what is spoken
        as the palate savours food?

12   There is wisdom, remember, in age,
        and long life brings understanding.)

---

[a] *Prob. rdg.; Heb. adds* and you will lie down unafraid.
doubt you are people.   [c] *Or* and he afflicted me.
adds He brings it in full measure to whom he will (*cp. 21. 17*).
posed to follow verse 12.

[b] *Prob. rdg.; Heb.* No
[d] *Prob. rdg.; Heb.*
[e] *Verse 10 trans-*

In God's hand are the souls of all that live,   10
the spirits of all human kind.
Wisdom and might are his,   13
with him are firmness and understanding.
If he pulls down, there is no rebuilding;   14
if he imprisons, there is no release.
If he holds up the waters, there is drought;   15
if he lets them go, they turn the land upside down.
Strength and success belong to him,   16
deceived and deceiver are his to use.
He makes counsellors behave like idiots   17
and drives judges mad;
he looses the bonds imposed by kings   18
and removes the girdle of office from their waists;
he makes priests behave like idiots   19
and overthrows men long in office;
those who are trusted he strikes dumb,   20
he takes away the judgement of old men;
he heaps scorn on princes   21
and abates the arrogance of nobles.
He leads peoples astray and destroys them,   23*a*
he lays them low, and there they lie.
He takes away their wisdom from the rulers of the nations   24
and leaves them wandering in a pathless wilderness;
they grope in the darkness without light   25
and are left to wander like a drunkard.
He uncovers mysteries deep in obscurity   22
and into thick darkness he brings light.

All this I have seen with my own eyes,   **13**
with my own ears I have heard it, and understood it.
What you know, I also know;   2
in nothing do I fall short of you.
But for my part I would speak with the Almighty   3
and am ready to argue with God,
while you like fools are smearing truth with your falsehoods, 4
stitching a patchwork of lies, one and all.
Ah, if you would only be silent   5
and let silence be your wisdom!
Now listen to my arguments   6
and attend while I put my case.
Is it on God's behalf that you speak so wickedly,   7
or in his defence that you allege what is false?
Must you take God's part,   8
or put his case for him?
Will all be well when he examines you?   9
Will you quibble with him as you quibble with a man?

a   Verse 22 transposed to follow verse 25.

xxvii

10 He will most surely expose you
    if you take his part by falsely accusing me.
11 Will not God's majesty strike you with dread,
    and terror of him overwhelm you?
12 Your pompous talk is dust and ashes,
    your defences will crumble like clay.
13 Be silent, leave me to speak my mind,
    and let what may come upon me!
14 I will put my neck in the noose
    and take my life in my hands.
15 If he would slay me, I should not hesitate;
    I should still argue my cause to his face.
16 This at least assures my success,
    that no godless man may appear before him.
17 Listen then, listen to my words,
    and give a hearing to my exposition.
18 Be sure of this: once I have stated my case
    I know that I shall be acquitted.
19 Who is there that can argue so forcibly with me
    that he could reduce me straightway to silence and death?

20 Grant me these two conditions only,
    and then I will not hide myself out of thy sight:
21 take thy heavy hand clean away from me
    and let not the fear of thee strike me with dread.
22 Then summon me, and I will answer;
    or I will speak first, and do thou answer me.
23 How many iniquities and sins are laid to my charge?
    let me know my offences and my sin.
24 Why dost thou hide thy face
    and treat me as thy enemy?
25 Wilt thou chase a driven leaf,
    wilt thou pursue dry chaff,
26 prescribing punishment for me
    and making me heir to the iniquities of my youth,
27 putting my feet in the stocks *a*
    and setting a slave-mark on the arches of my feet? *b*

14 Man born of woman is short-lived and full of disquiet.
 2 He blossoms like a flower and then he withers;
    he slips away like a shadow and does not stay;
    c he is like a wine-skin that perishes
    or a garment that moths have eaten.
 3 Dost thou fix thine eyes on such a creature,
    and wilt thou bring him into court to confront thee? *d*

---

a *Prob. rdg.; Heb. adds* keeping a close watch on all I do.   *b* *Prob. rdg.; Heb. adds*
verse 28, he is like . . . have eaten, *now transposed to follow 14. 2.*   *c* he is like . . .
have eaten: *13. 28 transposed here.*   *d* *So one Heb. MS.; others add* (4) Who can
produce pure out of unclean? No one.

The days of his life are determined,   5
and the number of his months is known to thee;
thou hast laid down a limit, which he cannot pass.
Look away from him therefore and leave him alone   6
counting the hours day by day like a hired labourer.

If a tree is cut down,   7
there is hope that it will sprout again
and fresh shoots will not fail.
Though its roots grow old in the earth,   8
and its stump is dying in the ground,
if it scents water it may break into bud   9
and make new growth like a young plant.
But a man dies, and he disappears;*a*   10
man comes to his end, and where is he?
As the waters of a lake dwindle,   11
or as a river shrinks and runs dry,
so mortal man lies down, never to rise   12
until the very sky splits open.
If a man dies, can he live again?*b*
He shall never be roused from his sleep.
If only thou wouldst hide me in Sheol   13
and conceal me till thy anger turns aside,
if thou wouldst fix a limit for my time there, and then remember me!
*c*Then I would not lose hope, however long my service,   14
waiting for my relief to come.
Thou wouldst summon me, and I would answer thee;   15
thou wouldst long to see the creature thou hast made.
But now thou dost count every step I take,   16
watching all my course.
Every offence of mine is stored in thy bag;   17
thou dost keep my iniquity under seal.
Yet as a falling mountain-side is swept away,   18
and a rock is dislodged from its place,
as water wears away stones,   19
and a rain-storm scours the soil from the land,
so thou hast wiped out the hope of frail man;
thou dost overpower him finally, and he is gone;   20
his face is changed, and he is banished from thy sight.
His flesh upon him becomes black,   22 *d*
and his life-blood dries up within him.*e*
His sons rise to honour, and he sees nothing of it;   21
they sink into obscurity, and he knows it not.

a Or *and is powerless.*   *b* *Line transposed from beginning of verse 14.*   *c* *See note
on verse 12.*   *d* *Verses 21 and 22 transposed.*   *e* *His flesh . . . within him:* or
His own kin, maybe, regret him, and his slaves mourn his loss.

Second cycle of speeches

15 Then Eliphaz the Temanite answered:

2 Would a man of sense give vent to such foolish notions
and answer with a bellyful of wind?

3 Would he bandy useless words
and arguments so unprofitable?

4 Why! you even banish the fear of God from your mind,
usurping the sole right to speak in his presence;

5 your iniquity dictates what you say,
and deceit is the language of your choice.

6 You are condemned out of your own mouth, not by me;
your own lips give evidence against you.

7 Were you born first of mankind?
were you brought forth before the hills?

8 Do you listen in God's secret council
or usurp all wisdom for yourself alone?

9 What do you know that we do not know?
What insight have you that we do not share?

10 We have age and white hairs in our company,
men older than your father.

11 Does not the consolation of God suffice you,
a word whispered quietly in your ear?

12 What makes you so bold at heart,
and why do your eyes flash,

13 that you vent your anger on God
and pour out such a torrent of words?

14 What is frail man that he should be innocent,
or any child of woman that he should be justified?

15 If God puts no trust in his holy ones,
and the heavens are not innocent in his sight,

16 how much less so is man, who is loathsome and rotten
and laps up evil like water!

17 I will tell you, if only you will listen,
and I will describe what I have seen

18 [what has been handed down by wise men
and was not concealed from them by their fathers;

19 to them alone the land was given,
and no foreigner settled among them]:

20 the wicked are racked with anxiety all their days,
the ruthless man for all the years in store for him.

21 The noise of the hunter's scare rings in his ears,
and in time of peace the raider falls on him;

22 he cannot hope to escape from dark death;
he is marked down for the sword;

he is flung out as food for vultures;   23
such a man knows that his destruction is certain.
Suddenly a black day comes upon him,   24
distress and anxiety overwhelm him
[like a king ready for battle];
for he has lifted his hand against God   25
and is pitting himself against the Almighty,
charging him head down,   26
with the full weight of his bossed shield.

Heavy though his jowl is and gross,   27
and though his sides bulge with fat,
the city where he lives will lie in ruins,   28
his house will be deserted;
it will soon become a heap of rubble.
He will no longer be rich, his wealth will not last,   29
and he will strike no root in the earth; *a*
scorching heat will shrivel his shoots,   30
and his blossom will be shaken off by the wind.
He deceives himself, trusting in his high rank,   31
for all his dealings will come to nothing.
His palm-trees will wither unseasonably,   32
and his branches will not spread;
he will be like a vine that sheds its unripe grapes,   33
like an olive-tree that drops its blossom.
For the godless, one and all, are barren,   34
and their homes, enriched by bribery, are destroyed by fire;
they conceive mischief and give birth to trouble,   35
and the child of their womb is deceit.

Then Job answered: **16**

I have heard such things often before,   2
you who make trouble, all of you, with every breath,
saying, 'Will this windbag never have done?   3
What makes him so stubborn in argument?'
If you and I were to change places,   4
I could talk like you;
how I could harangue you
and wag my head at you!
But no, I would speak words of encouragement,   5
and then my condolences would flow in streams.
If I speak, my pain is not eased;   6
if I am silent, it does not leave me.
Meanwhile, my friend wearies me with false sympathy;   7
they tear me to pieces, he and his *b* fellows.   8
He has come forward to give evidence against me;

---

a *Prob. rdg.; Heb. adds* he will not escape from darkness.   *b* *Prob. rdg.; Heb.* my.

the liar testifies against me to my face,
9   in his wrath he wears me down, his hatred is plain to see;
he grinds his teeth at me.

My enemies look daggers at me,
10   they bare their teeth to rend me,
they slash my cheeks with knives;
they are all in league against me.
11   God has left me at the mercy of malefactors
and cast me into the clutches of wicked men.
12   I was at ease, but he set upon me and mauled me,
seized me by the neck and worried me.
He set me up as his target;
13   his arrows rained upon me from every side;
pitiless, he cut deep into my vitals,
he spilt my gall on the ground.
14   He made breach after breach in my defences;
he fell upon me like a fighting man.

15   I stitched sackcloth together to cover my body
and I buried my forelock in the dust;
16   my cheeks were flushed with weeping
and dark shadows were round my eyes,
17   yet my hands were free from violence
and my prayer was sincere.

18   O earth, cover not my blood
and let my cry for justice find no rest!
19   For look! my witness is in heaven;
there is one on high ready to answer for me.
20   My appeal will come before God,
while my eyes turn again and again to him.
21   If only there were one to arbitrate between man and God,
as between a man and his neighbour!
22   For there are but few years to come
before I take the road from which I shall not return.

17   My mind is distraught, my days are numbered,
and the grave is waiting for me.
2   Wherever I turn, men taunt me,
and my day is darkened by their sneers.
3   Be thou my surety with thyself,
for who else can pledge himself for me?
4   Thou wilt not let those men triumph,
whose minds thou hast sunk in ignorance;
5   if such a man denounces his friends to their ruin,
his sons' eyes shall grow dim.

6   I am held up as a byword in every land,
a portent for all to see;

my eyes are dim with grief, 7
my limbs wasted to a shadow.
Honest men are bewildered at this, 8
and the innocent are indignant at my plight.
In spite of all, the righteous man maintains his course, 9
and he whose hands are clean grows strong again.

But come on, one and all, try again! 10
I shall not find a wise man among you.

My days die away like an echo; 11
my heart-strings *a* are snapped.
Day is turned into night, 12
and morning *b* light is darkened before me.
If I measure Sheol for my house, 13
if I spread my couch in the darkness,
if I call the grave my father 14
and the worm my mother or my sister,
where, then, will my hope be, 15
and who will take account of my piety?
I cannot take them down to Sheol with me, 16
nor can they descend with me into the earth.

Then Bildad the Shuhite answered: **18**

How soon will you bridle *c* your tongue? 2
Do but think, and then we will talk.
What do you mean by treating us as cattle? 3
Are we nothing but brute beasts to you? *d*
Is the earth to be deserted to prove you right, 4
or the rocks to be moved from their place?

No, it is the wicked whose light is extinguished, 5
from whose fire no flame will rekindle;
the light fades in his tent, 6
and his lamp dies down and fails him.
In his iniquity his steps totter, 7
and his disobedience trips him up;
he rushes headlong into a net 8
and steps through the hurdle that covers a pit;
his heel is caught in a snare, 9
the noose grips him tight;
a cord lies hidden in the ground for him 10
and a trap in the path.
The terrors of death suddenly beset him 11
and make him piss over his feet.

a Prob. rdg.; Heb. the desires of my heart. *b* morning: *prob. rdg.; Heb.* near.
c bridle: *prob. rdg.; Heb. unintelligible.* *d Prob. rdg.; Heb. adds* rending himself
in his anger.

12 For all his vigour he is paralysed with fear;
strong as he is, disaster awaits him.

13 Disease eats away his skin,
Death's eldest child devours his limbs.

14 He is torn from the safety of his home,
and Death's terrors escort him to their king. *a*

15 Magic herbs lie strewn about his tent,
and his home is sprinkled with sulphur to protect it.

16 His roots beneath dry up,
and above, his branches wither.

17 His memory vanishes from the face of the earth
and he leaves no name in the world.

18 He is driven from light into darkness
and banished from the land of the living.

19 He leaves no issue or offspring among his people,
no survivor in his earthly home;

20 in the west men hear of his doom and are appalled;
in the east they shudder with horror.

21 Such is the fate of the dwellings of evildoers,
and of the homes of those who care nothing for God.

19 Then Job answered:

2 How long will you exhaust me
and pulverize me with words?

3 Time and time again you have insulted me
and shamelessly done me wrong.

4 If in fact I had erred,
the error would still be mine.

5 But if indeed you lord it over me
and try to justify the reproaches levelled at me,

6 I tell you, God himself has put me in the wrong,
he has drawn the net round me.

7 If I cry 'Murder!' no one answers;
if I appeal for help, I get no justice.

8 He has walled in my path so that I cannot break away,
and he has hedged in the road before me.

9 He has stripped me of all honour
and has taken the crown from my head.

10 On every side he beats me down and I am gone;
he has pulled up my tent-rope *b* like a tree.

11 His anger is hot against me
and he counts me his enemy.

12 His raiders gather in force *c*
and encamp about my tent.

---

a Or and you conduct him to the king of terrors.   *b Or* he has uprooted my hope.
c Prob. rdg.; Heb. adds they raise an earthwork against me.

My brothers hold aloof from me,   13
my friends are utterly estranged from me;
my kinsmen and intimates fall away,   14-15
my retainers have forgotten me;
my slave-girls treat me as a stranger,
I have become an alien in their eyes.
I summon my slave, but he does not answer,   16
though I entreat him as a favour.
My breath is noisome to my wife,   17
and I stink in the nostrils of my own family.
Mere children despise me   18
and, when I rise, turn their backs on me;
my intimate companions loathe me,   19
and those whom I love have turned against me.
My bones stick out through my skin,*a*   20
and I gnaw my under-lip with my teeth.

Pity me, pity me, you that are my friends;   21
for the hand of God has touched me.
Why do you pursue me as God pursues me?   22
Have you not had your teeth in me long enough?
O that my words might be inscribed,   23
O that they might be engraved in an inscription,
cut with an iron tool and filled with lead   24
to be a witness*b* in hard rock!
But in my heart I know that my vindicator lives   25
and that he will rise last to speak in court;
and I shall discern my witness standing at my side*c*   26
and see my defending counsel, even God himself,
whom I shall see with my own eyes,   27
I myself and no other.

My heart failed me when you said,   28
'What a train of disaster he has brought on himself!
The root of the trouble lies in him.'
Beware of the sword that points at you,   29
the sword that sweeps away all iniquity;
then you will know that there is a judge.*d*

Then Zophar the Naamathite answered: **20**

My distress of mind forces me to reply,   2
and this is why*e* I hasten to speak:
I have heard arguments that are a reproach to me,   3
a spirit beyond my understanding gives me the answers.

---

a *Prob. rdg.; Heb. adds* and my flesh.   *b* to . . . witness: *or* for ever.   *c* my
witness . . . side: *prob. rdg.; Heb. unintelligible.*   *d* *Or* judgement.   *e* this is
why: *prob. rdg.; Heb. obscure.*

4   Surely you know that this has been so since time began,
      since man was first set on the earth:

5   the triumph of the wicked is short-lived,
      the glee of the godless lasts but a moment?

6   Though he stands high as heaven,
      and his head touches the clouds,

7   he will be swept utterly away like his own dung,
      and all that saw him will say, 'Where is he?'

8   He will fly away like a dream and be lost,
      driven off like a vision of the night;

9   the eye which glimpsed him shall do so no more
      and shall never again see him in his place.

11[a]   The youth and strength which filled his bones
      shall lie with him in the dust.

10   His sons will pay court to the poor,
      and their[b] hands will give back his wealth.

12   Though evil tastes sweet in his mouth,
      and he savours it, rolling it round his tongue,

13   though he lingers over it and will not let it go,
      and holds it back on his palate,

14   yet his food turns in his stomach,
      changing to asps' venom within him.

15   He gulps down wealth, then vomits it up,
      or God makes him discharge it.

16   He sucks the poison of asps,
      and the tongue of the viper kills him.

17   Not for him to swill down rivers of cream[c]
      or torrents of honey and curds;

18   he must give back his gains without swallowing them,
      and spew up his profit undigested;

19   for he has hounded and harassed the poor,
      he has seized houses which he did not build.

20   Because his appetite gave him no rest,
      and he cannot escape his own desires,

21   nothing is left for him to eat,
      and so his well-being does not last;

22   with every need satisfied his troubles begin,
      and the full force of hardship strikes him.

23   God vents his anger upon him
      and rains on him cruel blows.

24   He is wounded by weapons of iron
      and pierced by a bronze-tipped arrow;

25   out at his back the point comes,
      the gleaming tip from his gall-bladder.

26   Darkness unrelieved awaits him,
      a fire that needs no fanning will consume him.

[a] *Verses 10 and 11 transposed.*   [b] *Prob. rdg.; Heb. his.*   [c] rivers of cream:
prob. rdg.; Heb. obscure.

[Woe betide any survivor in his tent!]
The heavens will lay bare his guilt, 27
and earth will rise up to condemn him.
A flood will sweep away his house, 28
rushing waters on the day of wrath.
Such is God's reward for the wicked man 29
and the lot appointed for the rebel*a* by God.

Then Job answered: **21**

Listen to me, do but listen, 2
and let that be the comfort you offer me.
Bear with me while I have my say; 3
when I have finished, you may mock.
May not I too voice*b* my thoughts? 4
Have not I as good cause to be impatient?
Look at my plight, and be aghast; 5
clap your hand to your mouth.
When I stop to think, I am filled with horror, 6
and my whole body is convulsed.

Why do the wicked enjoy long life, 7
hale in old age, and great and powerful?
They live to see their children settled, 8
their kinsfolk and descendants flourishing;
their families are secure and safe; 9
the rod of God's justice does not reach them.
Their bull mounts and fails not of its purpose; 10
their cow calves and does not miscarry.
Their children like lambs run out to play, 11
and their little ones skip and dance;
they rejoice with tambourine and harp 12
and make merry to the sound of the flute.
Their lives close in prosperity, 13
and they go down to Sheol in peace.
To God they say, 'Leave us alone; 14
we do not want to know your ways.
What is the Almighty that we should worship him, 15
or what should we gain by seeking his favour?'

Is not the prosperity of the wicked in their own hands? 16
Are not their purposes very different from God's*c*?
How often is the lamp of the wicked snuffed out, 17
and how often does their ruin come upon them?
How often does God in his anger deal out suffering,
bringing it in full measure to whom he will?*d*

---

a the rebel: *prob. rdg.; Heb.* hiṣ word. *b* May . . . voice: *prob. rdg.; Heb. obscure.*
c God's: *prob. rdg.; Heb.* mine. *d* *Line transposed from 12. 6.*

18 How often is that man like a wisp of straw before the wind,
    like chaff which the storm-wind whirls away?
19 You say, 'The trouble he has earned, God will keep for his
        sons';
    no, let him be paid for it in full and be punished.
20 Let his own eyes see damnation come upon him,
    and the wrath of the Almighty be the cup he drinks.
21 What joy shall he have in his children after him,
    if his very months and days are numbered?
22 Can any man teach God,
    God who judges even those in heaven above?

23 One man, I tell you, dies crowned with success,
    lapped in security and comfort,
24 his loins full of vigour
    and the marrow juicy in his bones;
25 another dies in bitterness of soul
    and never tastes prosperity;
26 side by side they are laid in earth,
    and worms are the shroud of both.

27 I know well what you are thinking
    and the arguments you are marshalling against me;
28 I know you will ask, 'Where is the great man's home now,
    what has become of the home of the wicked?'
29 Have you never questioned travellers?
    Can you not learn from the signs they offer,
30 that the wicked is spared when disaster comes
    and conveyed to safety before the day of wrath?
31 No one denounces his conduct to his face,
    no one requites him for what he has done.
32-33 When he is carried to the grave,
    all the world escorts him, before and behind;
    the dust of earth is sweet to him,
    and thousands keep watch at his tomb.
34 How futile, then, is the comfort you offer me!
    How false your answers ring!

Third cycle of speeches

22 Then Eliphaz the Temanite answered:

2   Can man be any benefit to God?
    Can even a wise man benefit him?
3   Is it an asset to the Almighty if you are righteous?
    Does he gain if your conduct is perfect?

Do not think that he reproves you because you are pious,   4
that on this count he brings you to trial.
No: it is because you are a very wicked man,   5
and your depravity passes all bounds.
Without due cause you take a brother in pledge,   6
you strip men of their clothes and leave them naked.
When a man is weary, you give him no water to drink   7
and you refuse bread to the hungry.
Is the earth, then, the preserve of the strong   8
and a domain for the favoured few?
Widows you have sent away empty-handed,   9
orphans you have struck defenceless.
No wonder that there are pitfalls in your path,   10
that scares are set to fill you with sudden fear.
The light is turned into darkness, and you cannot see;   11
the flood-waters cover you.
Surely God is at the zenith of the heavens   12
and looks down on all the stars, high as they are.
But you say, 'What does God know?   13
Can he see through thick darkness to judge?
His eyes cannot pierce the curtain of the clouds   14
as he walks to and fro on the vault of heaven.'
Consider the course of the wicked man,   15
the path the miscreant treads:
see how they are carried off before their time,   16
their very foundation flowing away like a river;
these men said to God, 'Leave us alone;   17
what can the Almighty do to us?'
Yet it was he that filled their houses with good things,   18
although their purposes and his were very different.
The righteous see their fate and exult,   19
the innocent make game of them;
for their riches are swept away,   20
and the profusion of their wealth is destroyed by fire.

Come to terms with God and you will prosper;   21
that is the way to mend your fortune.
Take instruction from his mouth   22
and store his words in your heart.
If you come back to the Almighty in true sincerity,   23
if you banish wrongdoing from your home,
if you treat your precious metal as dust *a*   24
and the gold of Ophir as stones from the river-bed,
then the Almighty himself will be your precious metal;   25
he will be your silver in double measure.
Then, with sure trust in *b* the Almighty,   26
you will raise your face to God;

a Prob. rdg.; Heb. if you put your precious metal on dust.   *b* with . . . in: *or* delighting in.

27   you will pray to him, and he will hear you,
       and you will have cause to fulfil your vows.
28   In all your designs you will succeed,
       and light will shine on your path;
29   but God brings down the pride of the haughty *a*
       and keeps safe the man of modest looks.
30   He will deliver the innocent, *b*
       and you will be delivered, because your hands are clean.

23 Then Job answered:
2   My thoughts today are resentful,
       for God's hand is heavy on me in my trouble.
3   If only I knew how to find him,
       how to enter his court,
4   I would state my case before him
       and set out my arguments in full;
5   then I should learn what answer he would give
       and find out what he had to say.
6   Would he exert his great power to browbeat me?
       No; God himself would never bring a charge against me.
7   There the upright are vindicated before him,
       and I shall win from my judge an absolute discharge.
8   If I go forward, *c* he is not there;
       if backward, *d* I cannot find him;
9   when I turn *e* left, *f* I do not descry him;
       I face right, *g* but I see him not.
10   But he knows me in action or at rest;
       when he tests me, I prove to be gold.
11   My feet have kept to the path he has set me,
       I have followed his way and not turned from it.
12   I do not ignore the commands that come from his lips,
       I have stored in my heart what he says.
13   He decides, *h* and who can turn him from his purpose?
       He does what his own heart desires.
14   What he determines, that he carries out;
       his mind is full of plans like these.
15   Therefore I am fearful of meeting him;
       when I think about him, *i* I am afraid;
16   it is God who makes me faint-hearted
       and the Almighty who fills me with fear,
17   yet I am not reduced to silence by the darkness
       nor *j* by the mystery which hides him.

---

a but . . . haughty: *prob. rdg.; Heb.* obscure.   *b* *Prob. rdg.; Heb.* the not innocent.
c Or east.   *d* Or west.   *e* *Prob. rdg.; Heb.* he turns.   *f* Or north.   *g* Or south.
h He decides: *prob. rdg.; Heb.* He in one.   *i* when . . . him: *or* I stand aloof.
j yet I am not . . . nor: *or* indeed I am . . . and . . .

^aThe day of reckoning is no secret to the Almighty,   24
though those who know him have no hint of its date.
Wicked men move boundary-stones   2
and carry away flocks and their shepherds.
In the field they reap what is not theirs,   6^b
and filch the late grapes from the rich^c man's vineyard.
They drive off the orphan's ass   3
and lead away the widow's ox with a rope.
They snatch the fatherless infant from the breast   9
and take the poor man's child in pledge.
They jostle the poor out of the way;   4
the destitute huddle together, hiding from them.
The poor rise early like the wild ass,   5
when it scours the wilderness for food;
but though they work till nightfall,^d
their children go hungry.^e
Naked and bare they pass the night;   7
in the cold they have nothing to cover them.
They are drenched by rain-storms from the hills   8
and hug the rock, their only shelter.
Naked and bare they go about their work,   10
and hungry they carry the sheaves;
they press the oil in the shade where two walls meet,   11
they tread the winepress but themselves go thirsty.
Far from the city, they groan like dying men,   12
and like wounded men they cry out;
but God pays no heed to their prayer.
Some there are who rebel against the light of day,   13
who know nothing of its ways
and do not linger in the paths of light.
The murderer rises before daylight   14
to kill some miserable wretch.^f
The seducer watches eagerly for twilight,   15
thinking, 'No eye will catch sight of me.'
The thief prowls^g by night,^h
his face covered with a mask,
and in the darkness breaks into houses   16
which he has marked down in the day.
One and all,ⁱ they are strangers to the daylight,
but dark night is morning to them;   17
and in the welter of night they are at home.
Such men are scum on the surface of the water;   18
their fields have a bad name throughout the land,
and no labourer will go near their vineyards.

^a *Prob. rdg.; Heb. prefixes* Why.   ^b *Verses 3-9 re-arranged to restore the natural order.*
^c *Or* wicked.   ^d *Prob. rdg.; Heb.* Arabah.   ^e go hungry: *prob. rdg.; Heb.* to it food.
^f *See note on verse 15.*   ^g The thief prowls: *prob. rdg.; Heb.* Let him be like a thief.   ^h *Line transposed from end of verse 14.*   ⁱ One and all: *transposed from after* but *in next verse.*

19   As drought and heat make away with snow,
     so the waters of Sheol*a* make away with the sinner.
20   The womb forgets him, the worm sucks him dry;
     he will not be remembered ever after. *b*
21   He may have wronged the barren childless woman
     and been no help to the widow;
22   yet God in his strength carries off even the mighty;
     they may rise, but they have no firm hope of life.
23   He lulls them into security and confidence;
     but his eyes are fixed on their ways.
24   For a moment they rise to the heights, but are soon gone;
     iniquity is snapped like a stick. *c*
     They are laid low and wilt like a mallow-flower;
     they droop like an ear of corn on the stalk.
25   If this is not so, who will prove me wrong
     and make nonsense of my argument?

25 Then Bildad the Shuhite answered:

2   Authority and awe rest with him
     who has established peace in his realm on high.
3   His squadrons are without number;
     at whom will they not spring from ambush?
4   How then can a man be justified in God's sight,
     or one born of woman be innocent?
5   If the circling moon is found wanting,
     and the stars are not innocent in his eyes,
6   much more so man who is but a maggot,
     mortal man who is only a worm.

26 Then Job answered:

2   What help you have given to the man without resource,
     what deliverance you have brought to the powerless!
3   What counsel you offer to a man at his wit's end,
     what sound advice to the foolish!
4   Who has prompted you to say such things,
     and whose spirit is expressed in your speech?

5   In the underworld the shades writhe in fear,
     the waters and all that live in them are struck with terror. *d*
6   Sheol is laid bare,
     and Abaddon uncovered before him.
7   God spreads the canopy of the sky over chaos
     and suspends earth in the void.
8   He keeps the waters penned in dense cloud-masses,
     and the clouds do not burst open under their weight.

a snow ... Sheol: *prob. rdg.; Heb.* snow-water, Sheol.   *b Prob. rdg.; Heb. here*
adds iniquity is snapped like a stick (*see note on verse 24*).   *c Line transposed from*
end of verse 20.   *d* are struck with terror: *prob. rdg.; Heb. om.*

He covers the face of the full moon,[a]   9
unrolling his clouds across it.
He has fixed the horizon on the surface of the waters   10
at the farthest limit of light and darkness.
The pillars of heaven quake   11
and are aghast at his rebuke.
With his strong arm he cleft the sea-monster,   12
and struck down the Rahab by his skill.
At his breath the skies are clear,   13
and his hand breaks the twisting[b] sea-serpent.
These are but the fringe of his power;   14
and how faint the whisper that we hear of him!
[Who could fathom the thunder of his might?]

Then Job resumed his discourse: 27

I swear by God, who has denied me justice,   2
and by the Almighty, who has filled me with bitterness:
so long as there is any life left in me   3
and God's breath is in my nostrils,
no untrue word shall pass my lips   4
and my tongue shall utter no falsehood.
God forbid that I should allow you to be right;   5
till death, I will not abandon my claim to innocence.
I will maintain the rightness of my cause, I will never give up;   6
so long as I live, I will not change.

May my enemy meet the fate of the wicked,   7
and my antagonist the doom of the wrongdoer!
What hope has a godless man, when he is cut off,[c]   8
when God takes away his life?
Will God listen to his cry   9
when trouble overtakes him?
Will he trust himself to the Almighty   10
and call upon God at all times?

I will teach you what is in God's power,   11
I will not conceal the purpose of the Almighty.
If all of you have seen these things,   12
why then do you talk such empty nonsense?

This is the lot prescribed by God for the wicked,   13
and the ruthless man's reward from the Almighty.
He may have many sons, but they will fall by the sword,   14
and his offspring will go hungry;
the survivors will be brought to the grave by pestilence,   15
and no widows will weep for them.

[a] *Or* He overlays the surface of his throne.   [b] *Or* primeval.   [c] *Or* What
is a godless man's thread of life when it is cut . . .

16   He may heap up silver like dirt
       and get himself piles of clothes;

17   he may get them, but the righteous will wear them,
       and his silver will be shared among the innocent.

18   The house he builds is flimsy as a bird's nest
       or a shelter put up by a watchman.

19   He may lie down rich one day, but never again;
       he opens his eyes and all is gone.

20   Disaster overtakes him like a flood,
       and a storm snatches him away in the night;

21   the east wind lifts him up and he is gone;
       it whirls him far from home;

22   it flings itself on him without mercy,
       and he is battered and buffeted by its force;

23   it snaps its fingers at him
       and whistles over him wherever he may be.

God's unfathomable wisdom

28   There are mines for silver
       and places where men refine gold;

2   where iron is won from the earth
       and copper smelted from the ore;

3   the end of the seam lies in darkness,
       and it is followed to its farthest limit.[a]

4   Strangers cut the galleries;[b]
       they are forgotten as they drive forward far from men.[c]

5   While corn is springing from the earth above,
       what lies beneath is raked over like a fire,

6   and out of its rocks comes lapis lazuli,
       dusted with flecks of gold.

7   No bird of prey knows the way there,
       and the falcon's keen eye cannot descry it;

8   proud beasts do not set foot on it,
       and no serpent comes that way.

9   Man sets his hand to the granite rock
       and lays bare the roots of the mountains;

10   he cuts galleries in the rocks,
       and gems of every kind meet his eye;

11   he dams up the sources of the streams
       and brings the hidden riches of the earth to light.

12   But where can wisdom be found?
       And where is the source of understanding?

13   No man knows the way to it;
       it is not found in the land of living men.

[a] *Prob. rdg.; Heb. adds* stones of darkness and deep darkness. [b] Strangers . . . galleries: *prob. rdg.; Heb. obscure.*   [c] *Prob. rdg.; Heb. adds* languishing without foothold.

The depths of ocean say, 'It is not in us',   14
and the sea says, 'It is not with me.'
Red gold cannot buy it,   15
nor can its price be weighed out in silver;
it cannot be set in the scales against gold of Ophir,   16
against precious cornelian or lapis lazuli;
gold and crystal are not to be matched with it,   17
no work in fine gold can be bartered for it;
black coral and alabaster are not worth mention,   18
and a parcel of wisdom fetches more than red coral;
topaz *ᵃ* from Ethiopia is not to be matched with it,   19
it cannot be set in the scales against pure gold.
Where then does wisdom come from,   20
and where is the source of understanding?
No creature on earth can see it,   21
and it is hidden from the birds of the air.
Destruction and death say,   22
'We know of it only by report.'
But God understands the way to it,   23
he alone knows its source;
for he can see to the ends of the earth   24
and he surveys everything under heaven.
When he made a counterpoise for the wind   25
and measured out the waters in proportion,
when he laid down a limit for the rain   26
and a path for the thunderstorm,
even then he saw wisdom and took stock of it,   27
he considered it and fathomed its very depths.
And he said to man: 28
    The fear of the Lord is wisdom,
    and to turn from evil is understanding.

Job's final survey of his case

Then Job resumed his discourse: **29**

If I could only go back to the old days,   2
to the time when God was watching over me,
when his lamp shone above my head,   3
and by its light I walked through the darkness!
If I could be as in the days of my prime,   4
when God protected my home,
while the Almighty was still there at my side,   5
and my servants stood round me,
while my path flowed with milk,   6
and the rocks streamed oil!

ᵃ Or chrysolite.

7   If I went through the gate out of the town
     to take my seat in the public square,
8   young men saw me and kept out of sight;
     old men rose to their feet,
9   men in authority broke off their talk
     and put their hands to their lips;
10   the voices of the nobles died away,
     and every man held his tongue.
21 *a* They listened to me expectantly
     and waited in silence for my opinion.
22   When I had spoken, no one spoke again;
     my words fell gently on them;
23   they waited for them as for rain
     and drank them in like showers in spring.
24   When I smiled on them, they took heart;
     when my face lit up, they lost their gloomy looks.
25   I presided over them, planning their course,
     like a king encamped with his troops. *b*

11   Whoever heard of me spoke in my favour,
     and those who saw me bore witness to my merit,
12   how I saved the poor man when he called for help
     and the orphan who had no protector.
13   The man threatened with ruin blessed me,
     and I made the widow's heart sing for joy.
14   I put on righteousness as a garment and it clothed me;
     justice, like a cloak or a turban, wrapped me round. *e*
15   I was eyes to the blind
     and feet to the lame;
16   I was a father to the needy,
     and I took up the stranger's cause.
17   I broke the fangs of the miscreant
     and rescued the prey from his teeth.
18   I thought, 'I shall die with my powers unimpaired
     and my days uncounted as the grains of sand, *c*
19   with my roots spreading out to the water
     and the dew lying on my branches,
20   with the bow always new in my grasp
     and the arrow ever ready to my hand.' *d*

30 But now I am laughed to scorn
     by men of a younger generation,
     men whose fathers I would have disdained
     to put with the dogs who kept my flock.
2   What use were their strong arms to me,
     since their sturdy vigour had wasted away?

---

a Verses 21-25 transposed to this point.   *b Prob. rdg.; Heb. adds as when one
comforts mourners.*   *c Or as those of the phoenix.*   *d Verses 21-25 transposed
to follow verse 10.*

They gnawed roots*a* in the desert,	3
gaunt with want and hunger,*b*	
they plucked saltwort and wormwood	4
and root of broom*c* for their food.	
Driven out from the society of men,*d*	5
pursued like thieves with hue and cry,	
they lived in gullies and ravines,	6
holes in the earth and rocky clefts;	
they howled like beasts among the bushes,	7
huddled together beneath the scrub,	
vile base-born wretches,	8
hounded from the haunts of men.	
Now I have become the target of their taunts,	9
my name is a byword among them.	
They loathe me, they shrink from me,	10
they dare to spit in my face.	
They run wild and savage*e* me;	11
at sight of me they throw off all restraint.	
On my right flank they attack in a mob;*f*	12
they raise their siege-ramps against me,	
they tear down my crumbling defences to my undoing,	13
and scramble up against me unhindered;	
they burst in through the gaping breach;	14
at the moment of the crash they come rolling in.	
Terror upon terror overwhelms me,	15
it sweeps away my resolution like the wind,	
and my hope of victory vanishes like a cloud.	
So now my soul is in turmoil within me,	16
and misery has me daily in its grip.	
By night pain pierces my very bones,	17
and there is ceaseless throbbing in my veins;	
my garments are all bespattered with my phlegm,	18
which chokes me like the collar of a shirt.	
God himself*g* has flung me down in the mud,	19
no better than dust or ashes.	
I call for thy help, but thou dost not answer;	20
I stand up to plead, but thou sittest aloof;	
thou hast turned cruelly against me	21
and with thy strong hand pursuest me in hatred;	
thou dost snatch me up and set me astride the wind,	22
and the tempest*h* tosses me up and down.	
I know that thou wilt hand me over to death,	23
to the place appointed for all mortal men.	

a roots: *prob. rdg.; Heb. om.*   *b Prob. rdg.; Heb. adds* yesterday waste and derelict
land.   *c* root of broom: *probably* fungus on broom root.   *d* the society of men: *prob.
rdg.; Heb. obscure.*   *e* They run . . . savage: *prob. rdg.; Heb.* He runs . . . savages.
f Prob. rdg.; Heb. adds they let loose my feet.   *g* God himself: *prob. rdg.; Heb. om.*
h the tempest: *prob. rdg.; Heb. unintelligible.*

24 Yet no beggar held out his hand
    but was relieved*a* by me in his distress.
25 Did I not weep for the man whose life was hard?
    Did not my heart grieve for the poor?
26 Evil has come though I expected good;
    I looked for light but there came darkness.
27 My bowels are in ferment and know no peace;
    days of misery stretch out before me.
28 I go about dejected and friendless;
    I rise in the assembly, only to appeal for help.
29 The wolf is now my brother,
    the owls of the desert have become my companions.
30 My blackened skin peels off,
    and my body is scorched by the heat.
31 My harp has been tuned for a dirge,
    my flute to the voice of those who weep.

31 2*b* What is the lot prescribed by God above,
    the reward from the Almighty on high?
3   Is not ruin prescribed for the miscreant
    and calamity for the wrongdoer?
4   Yet does not God himself see my ways
    and count my every step?

5   I swear I have had no dealings with falsehood
    and have not embarked on a course of deceit.
1   I have come to terms with my eyes,
    never to take notice of a girl.
6   Let God weigh me in the scales of justice,
    and he will know that I am innocent!
7   If my steps have wandered from the way,
    if my heart has followed my eyes,
    or any dirt stuck to my hands,
8   may another eat what I sow,
    and may my crops be pulled up by the roots!
9   If my heart has been enticed by a woman
    or I have lain in wait at my neighbour's door,
10 may my wife be another man's slave,
    and may other men enjoy her.
11 [But that is a wicked act, an offence before the law;
12 it would be a consuming and destructive fire,
    raging *c* among my crops.]
13 If I have ever rejected the plea of my slave
    or of my slave-girl, when they brought their complaint to me,
14 what shall I do if God appears?
    What shall I answer if he intervenes?
15 Did not he who made me in the womb make them?

a was relieved: *prob. rdg.; Heb. unintelligible.*   *b* *Verse 1 transposed to follow verse 5.*
c *Prob. rdg.; Heb. uprooting.*

Did not the same God create us in the belly?
If I have withheld their needs from the poor   16
or let the widow's eye grow dim with tears,
if I have eaten my crust alone,   17
and the orphan has not shared it with me—
the orphan who from boyhood honoured me like a father,   18
whom I guided from the day of his*a* birth—
if I have seen anyone perish for lack of clothing,   19
or a poor man with nothing to cover him,
if his body had no cause to bless me,   20
because he was not kept warm with a fleece from my flock,
if I have raised*b* my hand against the innocent,*c*   21
knowing that men would side with me in court,
then may my shoulder-blade be torn from my shoulder,   22
my arm be wrenched out of its socket!
But the terror of God was heavy upon me,*d*   23
and for fear of his majesty I could do none of these things.
If I have put my faith in gold   24
and my trust in the gold of Nubia,
if I have rejoiced in my great wealth   25
and in the increase of riches;
if I ever looked on the sun in splendour   26
or the moon moving in her glory,
and was led astray in my secret heart   27
and raised my hand in homage;
this would have been an offence before the law,   28
for I should have been unfaithful to God on high.
If my land has cried out in reproach at me,   38*e*
and its furrows have joined in weeping,
if I have eaten its produce without payment   39
and have disappointed my creditors,
may thistles spring up instead of wheat,   40
and weeds instead of barley!

Have I rejoiced at the ruin of the man that hated me   29
or been filled with malice when trouble overtook him,
even though I did not allow my tongue to sin   30
by demanding his life with a curse?
Have the men of my household never said,   31
'Let none of us speak ill of him!
No stranger has spent the night in the street'?   32
For I have kept open house for the traveller.
Have I ever concealed my misdeeds as men do,   33
keeping my guilt to myself,
because I feared the gossip of the town   34
or dreaded the scorn of my fellow-citizens?

a *Prob. rdg.; Heb.* my.   *b* *Or* waved.   *c* *Or* orphan.   *d* *Prob. rdg.; Heb.* A fear towards me is a disaster from God.   *e* *Verses 38-40 transposed (but see note c, page 596).*

35   Let me but call a witness in my defence!
      Let the Almighty state his case against me!
      If my accuser had written out his indictment,
      I would not keep silence and remain indoors.*a*
36   No! I would flaunt it on my shoulder
      and wear it like a crown on my head;
37   I would plead the whole record of my life
      and present that in court as my defence.*b*

              Job's speeches are finished.*c*

Speeches of Elihu

32   So these three men gave up answering Job; for he continued to think him-
2   self righteous. Then Elihu son of Barakel the Buzite, of the family of Ram,
      grew angry; angry because Job had made himself out more righteous than
3   God,*d* and angry with the three friends because they had found no answer
4   to Job and had let God appear wrong.*e* Now Elihu had hung back while
5   they were talking with Job because they were older than he; but, when he
6   saw that the three had no answer, he could no longer contain his anger. So
      Elihu son of Barakel the Buzite began to speak:

          I am young in years,
          and you are old;
          that is why I held back and shrank
          from displaying my knowledge in front of you.
7   I said to myself, 'Let age speak,
          and length of years expound wisdom.'
8   But the spirit of God himself is in man,
          and the breath of the Almighty gives him understanding;
9   it is not only the old who are wise
          or the aged who understand what is right.
10   Therefore I say: Listen to me;
          I too will display my knowledge.
11   Look, I have been waiting upon your words,
          listening for the conclusions of your thoughts,
          while you sought for phrases;
12   I have been giving thought to your conclusions,
          but not one of you refutes Job or answers his arguments.
13   Take care then not to claim that you have found wisdom;
          God will rebut him, not man.
14   I will not string*f* words together like you*g*
          or answer him as you have done.

---

a Line transposed from verse 34.   *b Verses 38–40 transposed to follow verse 28 (but*
see note c).   *c The last line of verse 40 retained here.*   *d Or* had justified himself
with God.   *e Prob. original rdg., altered in Heb. to* and had not proved Job wrong.
f Prob. rdg.; Heb. He has not strung.   *g Prob. rdg.; Heb.* towards me.

If these men are confounded and no longer answer,   15
if words fail them,
am I to wait because they do not speak,   16
because they stand there and no longer answer?
I, too, have a furrow to plough;   17
I will express my opinion;
for I am bursting with words,   18
a bellyful of wind gripes me.
My stomach is distended as if with wine,   19
bulging like a blacksmith's bellows;
I must speak to find relief,   20
I must open my mouth and answer;
I will show no favour to anyone,   21
I will flatter no one, God or man;*a*
for I cannot use flattering titles,   22
or my Maker would soon do away with me.

Come now, Job, listen to my words   33
and attend carefully to everything I say.
Look, I am ready to answer;   2
the words are on the tip of my tongue.
My heart assures me that I speak with knowledge,   3
and that my lips speak with sincerity.
For the spirit of God made me,   4
and the breath of the Almighty gave me life.
Answer me if you can,   5
marshal your arguments and confront me.
In God's sight*b* I am just what you are;   6
I too am only a handful of clay.
Fear of me need not abash you,   7
nor any pressure from me overawe you.
You have said your say and I heard you;   8
I have listened to the sound of your words:
'I am innocent', you said, 'and free from offence,   9
blameless and without guilt.
Yet God finds occasions to put me in the wrong   10
and counts me his enemy;
he puts my feet in the stocks   11
and keeps a close watch on all I do.'

Well, this is my answer: You are wrong.   12
God is greater than man;
why then plead your case with him?   13
for no one can answer his arguments.
Indeed, once God has spoken   14
he does not speak a second time to confirm it.

---

a *Prob. rdg.; Heb.* I will not flatter man.   *b* In God's sight: *or* In strength.

15 In dreams, in visions of the night,
    when deepest sleep falls upon men,
16 while they sleep on their beds, God makes them listen,
    and his correction strikes them with terror.
17 To turn a man from reckless conduct,
    to check the pride*a* of mortal man,
18 at the edge of the pit he holds him back alive
    and stops him from crossing the river of death.
19 Or again, man learns his lesson on a bed of pain,
    tormented by a ceaseless ague in his bones;
20 he turns from his food with loathing
    and has no relish for the choicest meats;
21 his flesh hangs loose upon him,
    his bones are loosened and out of joint,
22 his soul draws near to the pit,
    his life to the ministers of death.
23 Yet if an angel, one of thousands, stands by him,
    a mediator between him and God,
    to expound what he has done right
    and to secure mortal man his due;*b*
24 if he speaks in the man's favour and says, 'Reprieve him,
    let him not go down to the pit, I have the price of his release';
25 then that man will grow sturdier*c* than he was in youth,
    he will return to the days of his prime.
26 If he entreats God to show him favour,
    to let him see his face and shout for joy;*d*
27 if he declares before all men, 'I have sinned,
    turned right into wrong and thought nothing of it';
28 then he saves himself from going down to the pit,
    he lives and sees the light.
29 All these things God may do to a man,
    again and yet again,
30 bringing him back from the pit
    to enjoy the full light of life.

31 Listen, Job, and attend to me;
    be silent, and I myself will speak.
32 If you have any arguments, answer me;
    speak, and I would gladly find you proved right;
33 but if you have none, listen to me:
    keep silence, and I will teach you wisdom.

34 Then Elihu went on to say:
2   Mark my words, you wise men;
    you men of long experience, listen to me;
3   for the ear tests what is spoken
    as the palate savours food.

---

a the pride: *prob. rdg.; Heb. obscure.*   *b Line transposed from verse 26.*   *c* will
grow sturdier: *prob. rdg.; Heb. unintelligible.*   *d See note on verse 23.*

Let us then examine for ourselves what is right;   4
let us together establish the true good.
Job has said, 'I am innocent,   5
but God has deprived me of justice,
he has falsified my case;   6
my state is desperate, yet I have done no wrong.'
Was there ever a man like Job   7
with his thirst for irreverent talk,
choosing bad company to share his journeys,   8
a fellow-traveller with wicked men?
For he says that it brings a man no profit   9
to find favour with God.
But listen to me, you men of good sense.   10
   Far be it from God to do evil
   or the Almighty to play false!
For he pays a man according to his work   11
and sees that he gets what his conduct deserves.
The truth is, God does no wrong,   12
the Almighty does not pervert justice.
Who committed the earth to his keeping?   13
Who but he established the whole world?
If he were to turn his thoughts inwards   14
and recall his life-giving spirit,
all that lives would perish on the instant,   15
and man return again to dust.

Now Job, if you have the wit, consider this;   16
listen to the words I speak.
Can it be that a hater of justice holds the reins?   17
Do you disparage a sovereign whose rule is so fair,
who will say to a prince, 'You scoundrel', .   18
and call his magnates blackguards to their faces;
who does not show special favour to those in office   19
and thinks no more of rich than of poor?
All alike are God's creatures,
who may die in a moment, in the middle of the night;   20
at his touch the rich are no more,
and the mighty vanish though no hand is laid on them.
His eyes are on the ways of men,   21
and he sees every step they take;
there is nowhere so dark, so deep in shadow,   22
that wrongdoers may hide from him.
Therefore he repudiates all that they do;   25
he turns on them in the night, and they are crushed.
There are no appointed days for men   23
to appear before God for judgement.
He holds no inquiry, but breaks the powerful   24
and sets up others in their place.

26 [a] For their crimes he strikes them down [b]
        and makes them disgorge their bloated wealth, [c]
27   because they have ceased to obey him
        and pay no heed to his ways.
28   Then the cry of the poor reaches his ears,
        and he hears the cry of the distressed.
29-30   [Even if he is silent, who can condemn him?
        If he looks away, who can find fault?
        What though he makes a godless man king
        over a stubborn nation and all its people?]

31   But suppose you were to say to God,
        'I have overstepped the mark; I will do no more [d] mischief.
32   Vile wretch that I am, be thou my guide;
        whatever wrong I have done, I will do wrong no more.'
33   Will he, at these words, condone your rejection of him?
        It is for you to decide, not me:
        but what can you answer?
34   Men of good sense will say,
        any intelligent hearer will tell me,
35   'Job talks with no knowledge,
        and there is no sense in what he says.
36   If only Job could be put to the test once and for all
        for answers that are meant to make mischief!
37   He is a sinner and a rebel as well [e]
        with his endless ranting against God.'

35 Then Elihu went on to say:

2   Do you think that this is a sound plea
        or maintain that you are in the right against God?—
3   if you say, 'What would be the advantage to me?
        how much should I gain from sinning?'
4   I will bring arguments myself against you,
        you and your three friends.
5   Look up at the sky and then consider,
        observe the rain-clouds towering above you.
6   How does it touch him if you have sinned?
        However many your misdeeds, what does it mean to him?
7   If you do right, what good do you bring him,
        or what does he gain from you?
8   Your wickedness touches only men, such as you are;
        the right that you do affects none but mortal man.

9   Men will cry out beneath the burdens of oppression
        and call for help against the power of the great;

---

[a] *Verse 25 transposed to follow verse 22.*   [b] he strikes them down: *prob. rdg.; Heb. om.*
[c] *Or and chastises them where people see.*   [d] more: *prob. rdg.; Heb. obscure.*
[e] *Prob. rdg.; Heb. adds* between us it is enough.

but none of them asks, 'Where is God my Maker 10
who gives protection by night,
who grants us more knowledge than the beasts of the earth 11
and makes us wiser than the birds of the air?'
So, when they cry out, he does not answer, 12
because they are self-willed and proud.
All to no purpose! God does not listen, 13
the Almighty does not see.

The worse for you when you say, 'He does not see me'! 14
Humble yourself^a in his presence and wait for his word.
But now, because God does not grow angry and punish 15
and because he lets folly pass unheeded,
Job gives vent to windy nonsense 16
and makes a parade of empty words.

Then Elihu went on to say: 36

Be patient a little longer, and let me enlighten you; 2
there is still something more to be said on God's side.
I will search far and wide to support my conclusions, 3
as I defend the justice of my Maker.
There are no flaws in my reasoning; 4
before you stands one whose conclusions are sound.

God,^b I say, repudiates the high and^c mighty 5
and does not let the wicked prosper, 6
but allows the just claims of the poor and suffering;
he does not deprive the sufferer of his due.^d 7
Look at kings on their thrones:
when God gives them sovereign power, they grow arrogant.
Next you may see them loaded with fetters, 8
held fast in captives' chains:
he denounces their conduct to them, 9
showing how insolence and tyranny was their offence;
his warnings sound in their ears 10
and summon them to turn back from their evil courses.
If they listen to him, they spend^e their days in prosperity 11
and their years in comfort.
But, if they do not listen, they die, their lesson unlearnt, 12
and cross the river of death.
Proud men rage against him 13
and do not cry to him for help when caught in his toils;
so they die in their prime, 14
like male prostitutes,^f worn out.^g

---

^a Humble yourself: *prob. rdg.; Heb.* Judge. ^b *Prob. rdg.; Heb. adds* a mighty one
and not. ^c and: *prob. rdg.; Heb. om.* ^d deprive ... due: *or* withdraw his
gaze from the righteous. ^e *Prob. rdg.; Heb. adds* they end. ^f *Cp. Deut. 23. 17.*
^g worn out: *prob. rdg.; Heb. unintelligible.*

15 Those who suffer he rescues through suffering
    and teaches them by the discipline of affliction.

16 Beware, if you are tempted to exchange hardship for comfort,[a]
    for unlimited plenty spread before you, and a generous table;
17 if you eat your fill of a rich man's fare
    when you are occupied with the business of the law,
18 do not be led astray by lavish gifts of wine
    and do not let bribery warp your judgement.
19 Will that wealth of yours, however great, avail you,
    or all the resources of your high position?
21[b] Take care not to turn to mischief;
    for that is why you are tried by affliction.

20 Have no fear if in the breathless terrors of the night
    you see nations vanish where they stand.
22 God towers in majesty above us;
    who wields such sovereign power as he?
23 Who has prescribed his course for him?
    Who has said to him, 'Thou hast done wrong'?
24 Remember then to sing the praises of his work,
    as men have always sung them.
25 All men stand back from[c] him;
    the race of mortals look on from afar.
26 Consider; God is so great that we cannot know him;
    the number of his years is beyond reckoning.
27 He draws up drops of water from the sea[d]
    and distils rain from the mist he has made;
28 the rain-clouds pour down in torrents,[e]
    they descend in showers on mankind;
31 thus he sustains the nations
    and gives them food in plenty.
29 Can any man read the secret of the sailing clouds,
    spread like a carpet under[f] his pavilion?
30 See how he unrolls the mist across the waters,
    and its streamers[g] cover the sea.
32[h] He charges the thunderbolts with flame
    and launches them straight[i] at the mark;
33 in his anger he calls up the tempest,
    and the thunder is the herald of its coming.[j]
37 This too makes my heart beat wildly
    and start from its place.
2   Listen, listen to the thunder of God's voice
    and the rumbling of his utterance.

---

[a] for comfort: *prob. rdg.; Heb. om.*   [b] *Verses 20 and 21 transposed.*   [c] *Or gaze at.*
[d] from the sea: *prob. rdg.; Heb. om.*   [e] in torrents: *prob. rdg.; Heb.* which.   [f] spread
. . . under: *prob. rdg.; Heb.* crashing noises.   [g] its streamers: *prob. rdg.; Heb.* the
roots of.   [h] *Verse 31 transposed to follow verse 28.*   [i] and . . . straight: *prob. rdg.; Heb.*
and gives orders concerning it.   [j] in his anger . . . coming: *prob. rdg.; Heb. obscure.*

Under the vault of heaven he lets it roll,   3
and his lightning reaches the ends of the earth;
there follows a sound of roaring   4
as he thunders with the voice of majesty.*a*
God's voice is marvellous in its working;*b*   5
he does great deeds that pass our knowledge.
For he says to the snow, 'Fall to earth',   6
and to the rainstorms, 'Be fierce.'
And when his voice is heard,
the floods of rain pour down unchecked.*c*
He shuts every man fast indoors,*d*   7
and all men whom he has made must stand idle;
the beasts withdraw into their lairs   8
and take refuge in their dens.
The hurricane bursts from its prison,   9
and the rain-winds bring bitter cold;
at the breath of God the ice-sheet is formed,   10
and the wide waters are frozen hard as iron.
He gives the dense clouds their load of moisture,   11
and the clouds spread his mist abroad,
as they travel round in their courses,   12
steered by his guiding hand
to do his bidding
all over the habitable world.*e*

Listen, Job, to this argument;   14
stand still, and consider God's wonderful works.
Do you know how God assigns them their tasks,   15
how he sends light flashing from his clouds?
Do you know why the clouds hang poised overhead,   16
a wonderful work of his consummate skill,
sweating there in your stifling clothes,   17
when the earth lies sultry under the south wind?
Can you beat out the vault of the skies, as he does,   18
hard as a mirror of cast metal?
Teach us then what to say to him;   19
for all is dark, and we cannot marshal our thoughts.
Can any man dictate to God when he is*f* to speak?   20
or command him to make proclamation?
At one moment the light is not seen,   21
it is overcast with clouds and rain;
then the wind passes by and clears them away,
and a golden glow comes from the north.*g*   22

---

a *See note on verse 6.*   *b* *Prob. rdg.; Heb.* thundering.   *c* And when . . . unchecked:
prob. rdg.; some words in these lines transposed from verse 4.   *d* indoors: *prob. rdg.;*
Heb. obscure.   *e* *Prob. rdg.; Heb. adds* (13) whether he makes him attain the rod,
or his earth, or constant love.   *f* *Prob. rdg.; Heb.* I am.   *g* *Prob. rdg.; Heb. adds*
this refers to God, terrible in majesty.

23   But the Almighty we cannot find; his power is beyond our ken,
      and his righteousness not slow to do justice.
24   Therefore mortal men pay him reverence,
      and all who are wise look to him.

God's answer and Job's submission

38 Then the LORD answered Job out of the tempest:

2   Who is this whose ignorant words
      cloud my design in darkness?
3   Brace yourself and stand up like a man;
      I will ask questions, and you shall answer.
4   Where were you when I laid the earth's foundations?
      Tell me, if you know and understand.
5   Who settled its dimensions? Surely you should know.
      Who stretched his measuring-line over it?
6   On what do its supporting pillars rest?
      Who set its corner-stone in place,
7   when the morning stars sang together
      and all the sons of God shouted aloud?
8   Who watched over the birth of the sea,[a]
      when it burst in flood from the womb?—
9   when I wrapped it in a blanket of cloud
      and cradled it in fog,
10   when I established its bounds,
      fixing its doors and bars in place,
11   and said, 'Thus far shall you come and no farther,
      and here your surging waves shall halt.'[b]
12   In all your life have you ever called up the dawn
      or shown the morning its place?
13   Have you taught it to grasp the fringes of the earth
      and shake the Dog-star from its place;
14   to bring up the horizon in relief as clay under a seal,
      until all things stand out like the folds of a cloak,
15   when the light of the Dog-star is dimmed
      and the stars of the Navigator's Line go out one by one?
16   Have you descended to the springs of the sea
      or walked in the unfathomable deep?
17   Have the gates of death been revealed to you?
      Have you ever seen the door-keepers of the place of darkness?
18   Have you comprehended the vast expanse of the world?
      Come, tell me all this, if you know.
19   Which is the way to the home of light
      and where does darkness dwell?

[a] *Who . . . sea: prob. rdg.; Heb.* And he held back the sea with two doors.   [b] *Prob. rdg.; Heb.* here one shall set on your surging waves.

And can you then take each to its appointed bound   20
and escort it on its homeward path?
Doubtless you know all this; for you were born already,   21
so long is the span of your life!

Have you visited the storehouse of the snow   22
or seen the arsenal where hail is stored,
which I have kept ready for the day of calamity,   23
for war and for the hour of battle?
By what paths is the heat spread abroad   24
or the east wind carried far and wide over the earth?
Who has cut channels for the downpour   25
and cleared a passage for the thunderstorm,
for rain to fall on land where no man lives   26
and on the deserted wilderness,
clothing lands waste and derelict with green   27
and making grass grow on thirsty ground *a*?
Has the rain a father?   28
Who sired the drops of dew?
Whose womb gave birth to the ice,   29
and who was the mother of the frost from heaven,
which lays a stony cover over the waters   30
and freezes the expanse of ocean?
Can you bind the cluster of the Pleiades   31
or loose Orion's belt?
Can you bring out the signs of the zodiac in their season   32
or guide Aldebaran and its train?
Did you proclaim the rules that govern the heavens,   33
or determine the laws of nature on earth?
Can you command the dense clouds   34
to cover you with their weight of waters?
If you bid lightning speed on its way,   35
will it say to you, 'I am ready'?
Who put wisdom in depths of darkness   36
and veiled understanding in secrecy *b*?
Who is wise enough to marshal the rain-clouds   37
and empty the cisterns of heaven,
when the dusty soil sets hard as iron,   38
and the clods of earth cling together?
Do you hunt her prey for the lioness   39
and satisfy the hunger of young lions,
as they crouch in the lair   40
or lie in wait in the covert?
Who provides the raven with its quarry   41
when its fledglings croak *c* for lack of food?

---

a thirsty ground: *prob. rdg.; Heb.* source.   *b* secrecy: *prob. rdg.; Heb. word unknown.*
c *Prob. rdg.; Heb. adds* they cry to God.

39   Do you know when the mountain-goats are born
     or attend the wild doe when she is in labour?

2   Do you count the months that they carry their young
     or know the time of their delivery,

3   when they crouch down to open their wombs
     and bring their offspring to the birth,

4   when the fawns grow and thrive in the open forest,
     and go forth and do not return?

5   Who has let the wild ass of Syria range at will
     and given the wild ass of Arabia its freedom?—

6   whose home I have made in the wilderness
     and its lair in the saltings;

7   it disdains the noise of the city
     and is deaf to the driver's shouting;

8   it roams the hills as its pasture
     and searches for anything green.

9   Does the wild ox consent to serve you,
     does it spend the night in your stall?

10   Can you harness its strength *a* with ropes,
     or will it harrow the furrows *a* after you?

11   Can you depend on it, strong as it is,
     or leave your labour to it?

12   Do you trust it to come back
     and bring home your grain to the threshing-floor?

13   The wings of the ostrich are stunted; *b.*
     c her pinions and plumage are so scanty *d*

14   that she abandons her eggs to the ground,
     letting them be kept warm by the sand.

15   She forgets that a foot may crush them,
     or a wild beast trample on them;

16   she treats her chicks heartlessly as if they were not hers,
     not caring if her labour is wasted

17   (for God has denied her wisdom
     and left her without sense),

18   while like a cock she struts over the uplands,
     scorning both horse and rider.

19   Did you give the horse his strength?
     Did you clothe his neck with a mane?

20   Do you make him quiver like a locust's wings,
     when his shrill neighing strikes terror?

21   He shows his mettle as he paws and prances;
     he charges the armoured line with all his might.

22   He scorns alarms and knows no dismay;
     he does not flinch before the sword.

---

a Prob. rdg.; Heb. transposes strength *and* furrows.
Heb. unintelligible.   *c Prob. rdg.; Heb. prefixes* if.
or stork.

b are stunted: *prob. rdg.;*
d Prob. rdg.; Heb. godly

The quiver rattles at his side,   23
the spear and sabre flash.
Trembling with eagerness, he devours the ground   24
and cannot be held in when he hears the horn;
at the blast of the horn he cries 'Aha!'   25
and from afar he scents the battle.*
Does your skill teach the hawk to use its pinions   26
and spread its wings towards the south?
Do you instruct the vulture to fly high   27
and build its nest aloft?
It dwells among the rocks and there it lodges;   28
its station is a crevice in the rock;
from there it searches for food,   29
keenly scanning the distance,
that its brood may be gorged with blood;   30
and where the slain are, there the vulture is.
Can you pull out the whale* with a gaff   **41** 1*
or can you slip a noose round its tongue?
Can you pass a cord through its nose   2
or put a hook through its jaw?
Will it plead with you for mercy   3
or beg its life with soft words?
Will it enter into an agreement with you   4
to become your slave for life?
Will you toy with it as with a bird   5
or keep it on a string like a song-bird for your maidens?
Do trading-partners haggle over it   6
or merchants share it out?

Then the LORD said to Job: **40**

Is it for a man who disputes with the Almighty to be stubborn?   2
Should he that argues with God answer back?

And Job answered the LORD: 3

What reply can I give thee, I who carry no weight?   4
I put my finger to my lips.
I have spoken once and now will not answer again;   5
twice have I spoken, and I will do so no more.

Then the LORD answered Job out of the tempest: 6

Brace yourself and stand up like a man;   7
I will ask questions, and you shall answer.
Dare you deny that I am just   8
or put me in the wrong that you may be right?

---

a *Prob. rdg.; Heb. adds* the thunder of the captains and the shouting.   *b* *Or* Leviathan.
c *41. 1-6 (in Heb. 40. 25-30) transposed to this point.*

9   Have you an arm like God's arm,
    can you thunder with a voice like his?
10 Deck yourself out, if you can, in pride and dignity,
    array yourself in pomp and splendour;
11 unleash the fury of your wrath,
    look upon the proud man and humble him;
12 look upon every proud man and bring him low,
    throw down the wicked where they stand;
13 hide them in the dust together,
    and shroud them in an unknown grave.
14 Then I in my turn will acknowledge
    that your own right hand can save you.

15 Consider the chief of the beasts, the crocodile,*a*
    who devours cattle as if they were grass:*b*
16 what strength is in his loins!
    what power in the muscles of his belly!
17 His tail is rigid as*c* a cedar,
    the sinews of his flanks are closely knit,
18 his bones are tubes of bronze,
    and his limbs like bars of iron.
19 He is the chief of God's works,
    made to be a tyrant over his peers;*d*
20 for he takes*e* the cattle of the hills for his prey
    and in his jaws he crunches all wild beasts.
21 There under the thorny lotus he lies,
    hidden in the reeds and the marsh;
22 the lotus conceals him in its shadow,
    the poplars of the stream surround him.
23 If the river is in spate, he is not scared,
    he sprawls at his ease though the stream is in flood.
24 Can a man blind*f* his eyes and take him
    or pierce his nose with the teeth of a trap?
41 7*g* Can you fill his skin with harpoons
    or his head with fish-hooks?
8   If ever you lift your hand against him,
    think of the struggle that awaits you, and let be.

9   No, such a man is in desperate case,
    hurled headlong at the very sight of him.
10 How fierce he is when he is roused!
    Who is there to stand up to him?
11 Who has ever attacked him*h* unscathed?
    Not a man*i* under the wide heaven.

a chief . . . crocodile: *prob. rdg.; Heb.* beasts (behemoth) which I have made with you.
b cattle . . . grass: *prob. rdg.; Heb.* grass like cattle.   *c* *Or* He bends his tail like . . .
d *Prob. rdg.; Heb.* his sword.   *e* *Prob. rdg.; Heb.* they take.   *f* Can a man blind:
prob. rdg.; Heb. obscure.   *g* *Verses 1–6 transposed to follow 39. 30.*   *h* *Prob. rdg.;*
Heb. me.   *i* *Prob. rdg.; Heb.* He is mine.

I will not pass over in silence his limbs,   12
his prowess and the grace of his proportions.
Who has ever undone his outer garment   13
or penetrated his doublet of hide?
Who has ever opened the portals of his face?   14
for there is terror in his arching teeth.
His back^a is row upon row of shields,   15
enclosed in a wall ^b of flints;
one presses so close on the other   16
that air cannot pass between them,
each so firmly clamped to its neighbour   17
that they hold and cannot spring apart.
His sneezing sends out sprays of light,   18
and his eyes gleam like the shimmer of dawn.
Firebrands shoot from his mouth,   19
and sparks come streaming out;
his nostrils pour forth smoke   20
like a cauldron on a fire blown to full heat.
His breath sets burning coals ablaze,   21
and flames flash from his mouth.
Strength is lodged in his neck,   22
and untiring energy dances ahead of him.
Close knit is his underbelly,   23
no pressure will make it yield.
His heart is firm as a rock,   24
firm as the nether millstone.
When he raises himself, strong men^c take fright,   25
bewildered at the lashings of his tail.
Sword or spear, dagger or javelin,   26
if they touch him, they have no effect.
Iron he counts as straw,   27
and bronze as rotting wood.
No arrow can pierce him,   28
and for him sling-stones are turned into chaff;
to him a club is a mere reed,   29
and he laughs at the swish of the sabre.
Armoured beneath with jagged sherds,   30
he sprawls on the mud like a threshing-sledge.
He makes the deep water boil like a cauldron,   31
he whips up the lake like ointment in a mixing-bowl.
He leaves a shining trail behind him,   32
and the great river is like white hair in his wake.
He has no equal on earth;   33
for he is made quite without fear.
He looks down on all creatures, even the highest;   34
he is king over all proud beasts.

^a *Prob. rdg.; Heb.* pride.   ^b *Prob. rdg.; Heb.* seal.   ^c strong men: *or* leaders
or gods.

42   Then Job answered the LORD:

2   I know that thou canst do all things
and that no purpose is beyond thee.

3   But I have spoken of great things which I have not understood,
things too wonderful for me to know.[a]

5   I knew of thee then only by report,
but now I see thee with my own eyes.

6   Therefore I melt away;[b]
I repent in dust and ashes.

Epilogue

7   When the LORD had finished speaking to Job, he said to Eliphaz the Temanite, 'I am angry with you and your two friends, because you have not spoken

8   as you ought about me, as my servant Job has done. So now take seven bulls
and seven rams, go to my servant Job and offer a whole-offering for your-
selves, and he will intercede for you; I will surely show him favour by not
being harsh with you because you have not spoken as you ought about me,

9   as he has done.' Then Eliphaz the Temanite and Bildad the Shuhite and
Zophar the Naamathite went and carried out the LORD's command, and
the LORD showed favour to Job when he had interceded for his friends.

10   So the LORD restored Job's fortunes and doubled all his possessions.

11   · Then all Job's brothers and sisters and his former acquaintance came
and feasted with him in his home, and they consoled and comforted him for
all the misfortunes which the LORD had brought on him; and each of them

12   gave him a sheep[c] and a gold ring. Furthermore, the LORD blessed the
end of Job's life more than the beginning; and he had fourteen thousand
head of small cattle and six thousand camels, a thousand yoke of oxen and

13 14   as many she-asses. He had seven[d] sons and three daughters; and he named
his eldest daughter Jemimah, the second Keziah and the third Keren-

15   happuch. There were no women in all the world so beautiful as Job's
daughters; and their father gave them an inheritance with their brothers.

16   Thereafter Job lived another hundred and forty years, he saw his sons

17   and his grandsons to four generations, and died at a very great age.

[a] *Prob. rdg.; Heb. adds* (4) O listen, and let me speak; I will ask questions, and you shall
answer.   [b] *Or* despise myself.   [c] *Or* piece of money.   [d] *Or* fourteen.

CHAPTER 1

Perspectives on Job

THE Book of Job opens with the sentence, "There lived in the land of Uz a man of blameless and upright life named Job. . . ." This opening sentence carries a number of messages. "There lived a man" is equivalent to "Once upon a time"; "in the land of Uz" has been taken to mean an unspecified far-off land; and, although the Book is included in the Hebrew scriptures, it was the opinion of Moses Maimonides that Job was not necessarily a Jew. The story, therefore, is intended to have universal application in time and geographical location, and to be without limitation to any one religious culture. It is an allegory of the human situation, in which all men may participate in various ways according to the culture in which they live. Job is a Biblical Everyman, and, in this sense, figures among the host of archetypes and prototypes from which collective and individual experiences are derived, expressed, and understood. Alongside the myths of Prometheus, Oedipus, Ulysses, and Faust, and the many legends of semihistorical characters, where a search for truth is carried out within the context of trials and suffering, the story of Job finds its place as a representation of spiritual evolution, through physical and mental suffering, into a new identity.

In the twelfth century, Maimonides, a Jew who lived in Spain and wrote in Arabic, had referred to the general lessons which could be drawn from the Book of Job. Physician, philosopher, and Biblical commentator, he was responsible for a new tradition of theological interpretation and understanding of Hebrew literature. He refers to "the strange and wonderful Book of Job" whose "basis is a fiction, conceived for the purpose of explaining the different opinions which people hold on

Divine Providence". He goes on to say: "This fiction, however, is in so far different from other fictions that it includes profound ideas and great mysteries, removes great doubts, and reveals the most important truths."[1]

Froude in 1853 commented on the complexity of the wording of the Book of Job. He discussed the difficulties encountered by the English translators of the Authorized and Revised Versions, as evinced in

> . . . the number of words which they were obliged to insert in italics, and the doubtful renderings which they have suggested in the margin. One instance of this, in passing, we will notice in this place—it will be familiar to every one as the passage quoted at the opening of the English burial service, and adduced as one of the doctrinal proofs of the resurrection of the body: "I know that my Redeemer liveth, and that He shall stand at the latter *day* upon the earth; and *though*, after my skin *worms* destroy this body, yet in my flesh I shall see God." So this passage stands in the ordinary version. But the words in italics have nothing answering to them in the original—they were all added by the translators to fill out their interpretation. . . .[2]

Froude's example of the use of the additional words to convey a meaning understood by the translator within his own contemporary religious framework is given point by the difference in the New English Version of this passage. It reads:

> But in my heart I know that my vindicator lives
> and that he will rise last to speak in court;
> and I shall discern my witness standing at my side
> and see my defending counsel, even God himself,
> whom I shall see with my own eyes,
> I myself and no other.   (19: 25–27)

It would be difficult to interpret ideas about resurrection from this translation.

The point of this is that the meaning of the Bible, even without the words in italics, is filled out in each generation according to contemporary thought and contemporary interpretations of human attitudes and motivations. There is a truism that the Bible is written in the language of man. For many people the Bible carries something eternal and unchanging, but we must recognize that language itself alters according to the meanings

---

[1] Moses Maimonides (1168), *The Guide for the Perplexed*, trans. M. Friedlander (London: George Routledge & Sons, 1947), p. 296.

[2] J. A. Froude, *Short Studies on Great Subjects* (London: J. M. Dent & Sons, 1906), p. 79.

which people attach to its constituent words. We are free, therefore, to add new meanings to the Book of Job just as, for example, it is possible to offer a stage production of Hamlet which is obviously influenced by the Freudian account of the Oedipus complex. The difference between the renderings of the Authorized and Revised Versions and the New English Version of Job 19: 25–27 is a good illustration of the discrepancies of interpretation, according to the culture of the time. Every translation is an interpretation.

In Robert Burton's *Anatomy of Melancholy*, quotations from the Book of Job form part of the rich storehouse of illustrative material drawn from the religious, philosophical, and anecdotal writings from the Greek, Roman, and Judeo-Christian civilizations. He ruminates over the question, "Was Job or the devil the greater conqueror? Surely Job. The devil had his [Job's] goods: he [Job] sate on the muckhill and kept his good name."[3] Concerning Job's wife, who from the start was relegated to an inferior position, Robert Burton quotes an interpretation that she was spared by the devil in order to increase the extent and duration of Job's persecution.[4]

The anthropologist Meyer Fortes has used the story of Job in a study of West African religions.[5] He introduced concepts from the stories of Oedipus and Job to illustrate ideas about fate or destiny which were embodied in these religions:

> What is notable then is that they epitomize, poignantly and dramatically, two religious and ethical conceptions that seem to be mutually opposed in some respects but complementary in others. These ideas are associated with different cosmological doctrines about the universe, and different conceptions of the nature of man and his relations with supernatural powers. I think that they represent, in a clear paradigmatic form, two fundamental principles of religious thought and custom. The Oedipal principle is best summed up in the notion of Fate or Destiny, the Jobian principle in that of Supernatural Justice.[6]

In the religions of West African tribes there is the sense of a prenatal destiny that can not be changed. In the Oedipus story the various attempts to alter the destiny as foretold by the oracle became the means by which the tragedy was created.

[3] Robert Burton, *Anatomy of Melancholy* (1621), Part 2, Sec. 3, Memb. 3.
[4] *Ibid.*, Part 2, Sec. 2, Memb. 6, Subs. 3.
[5] Meyer Fortes, *Oedipus and Job in West African Religion* (Cambridge: Cambridge University Press, 1959).
[6] *Ibid.*, p. 11.

In Job there was a parallel attempt to control destiny (or Divine Justice) by the "right" behaviour. Destiny is sensed in the experience which relates human behaviour to the good or bad fortunes which God is seen to mete out as justice. This is destiny only in so far as the behaviour has a natural corollary, i.e. if there is an exact proportion between God's distribution of reward and punishment on the one hand and the goodness and badness of the behaviour on the other. The story of Job begins with a concept of this type of retributive justice, but the outcome of the Book is a challenge to that idea.

Meyer Fortes discusses Job's claims on God and asks:

> Is not God all-powerful so that he stands above all human norms of good and bad conduct and is not bound by a concept of justice founded on a rule of reciprocal obligation? . . . Man is not God's equal, and however virtuous he may feel himself to be, he cannot measure himself against God to disannul God's 'udgement and condemn Him in order to justify himself.
> It is when he realizes the import of this speech (Job 40: 8) that Job is saved.[7]

It is part of our thesis that Job was able to achieve a new level of maturity when he came to forego his challenge to God in moral terms and was able to look beyond the realm of ethics to a vaster conception of the universe and man's place in it.

A modern literary use of the Jobian theme appears in the play *J.B.* by Archibald Macleish. This deals with the Book of Job in a modern setting, where some of the original poetic mystery of the Bible story is interpreted through the medium of contemporary drama. Macleish's version differs to the extent to which he calls particular attention to the character of Job's wife, who is virtually ignored in the Bible story. In the text, Job's wife is not killed, she is not punished, nor is she described as suffering. The omission of reference to her suffering is astonishing. An explanation has been given that Satan sees her more as a possible ally than as a victim, and that she might be an instrument in weakening Job's steadfastness. This kind of explanation reveals an attitude which assumes that steadfastness is righteous and to be approved, and that Job's wife could erode his integrity. "Then his wife said to him, 'Are you still unshaken in your integrity? Curse God and die'" (2: 9). Here we could take the liberty of adding words which were not in the original text in order to fill out the meaning. She might well have said, "Curse God and die . . . *like a man,*

---

[7] Meyer Fortes, *Oedipus and Job in West African Religion*, p. 17.

and not a bloody saint!" Textual justification for this addition could be found in the dénouement where twice God tells Job to "Brace yourself and stand up like a man" (38: 3 and 40: 7).

In Macleish's *J.B.*, on the other hand, the wife, Sarah, calls attention to the fact that J.B. has no right to monopolize either the mourning of their children nor to insist upon the righteousness of God. Speaking of their dead children, she says:

>   They are
>   Dead and they were innocent: I will not
>   Let you sacrifice their deaths
>   To make injustice justice and God good!
> J.B.   (covering his face with his hands)
>   My heart beats. I cannot answer it.
> Sarah: If you buy quiet with their innocence—
>   Theirs or yours. . . .
>   I will not love you.
> J.B.   (softly)
>   I have no choice but to be guilty.
> Sarah: (her voice rising)
>   We have the choice to live or die
>   All of us. . . .
>   *Curse God and die.* . . .[8]

Sarah believes that we have the choice to judge the God whose actions we disapprove. But J.B. responds:

> We have no choice but to be guilty;
> God is unthinkable if we are innocent.[9]

For some people it is unthinkable to believe in a God who allows children to be born handicapped or retarded or young people to die. Job's reaction to the calamities that befall him is to view them as punishment that is exclusively his own. His denial of his wife's right to sin and to be punished is a denial of her separate existence. It is a denial of her rights in the life of her children and of her suffering in the loss of them. When Sarah asks, "Has pain no meaning?", she could have meant her labour pains. However important fatherhood might be, there can be no gainsaying the intimacy of the relationship of mother and child. The joint experience of

[8] Archibald Macleish, *J.B.* (Boston: Houghton Mifflin Company, 1956), p. 110.
[9] *Ibid.*, p. 111.

one another, beginning in the pregnancy, is endorsed during the pains and labour of the confinement. Other Bible stories stress the depth of this relationship which, in the Book of Job, is ignored. Furthermore, at no point does the Bible story recognize the enormity of using the lives of children for the testing of the virtue of the parent. This is paralleled in the Oedipus legend by the complete omission of any questioning of the right of the parents to put their infant to death in order to avert the prophecy.

In *J.B.*, Macleish permits Sarah to represent the challenge to the concept of a God whose justice depends upon the human acceptance of guilt:

> Sarah: Must we be guilty for Him?—bear
> The burden of the world's malevolence
> For Him who made the world?[10]

William Blake adds new dimensions to the interpretations of the Job story in his series of illustrations. These drawings have been studied by Marion Milner[11] who points out the creative aspects of the spiritual agony of Job as represented symbolically by Blake. She begins by calling attention to the fact that Job's face is identical with that of God. In fact, one could go a stage further and state that his entire appearance is an almost exact facsimile of God's. Job's initial greatness comes from his confidence that whatever he is or does reflects God himself, and the reflection of God's image in Job is so perfect that he is set above his family and his neighbours.

It is worth noting that in the picture which shows the messenger bringing the news of disasters (" ' and I am the only one to escape and tell the tale' "), the news is presented to Job and his wife together. Blake thus adds to the Bible text by depicting Job's wife sharing equally in the grief.

Milner goes on to develop the themes of Job's descent to the depths of suffering and his subsequent recovery. She suggests that his sense of wholeness was related to his own experience of being mothered:

> Naked I came from the womb,
> naked I shall return whence I came.
>   (1: 21)

---

[10] Archibald Macleash, *J. B.*, p. 109.

[11] Marion Milner, "The sense in non-sense—Freud and Blake's Job", *Freud, Jung and Adler: Their Relevance to the Teacher's Life and Work*, reprinted from *The New Era*, No. 1 (Jan. 1956), pp. 29–41.

She states that he now recognizes that he was helpless as an infant:

> . . . his initial feeling of wholeness,[12] unity with the universe, was only made possible because he had a mother there, separate from himself and therefore able to nourish and protect him from the hurtful impacts of that universe. But he does not yet recognize his anger at having eventually to give up both that protection and also the illusion that he did not need it because he thought he did it all himself. He does not yet recognize his anger, but his body breaks out in boils.[13]

During the process of recovery, Job began

> . . . to realize that his thoughts and wishes are not omnipotent and therefore that he is not responsible for everything that happens, either for good or for evil.[14]

Marion Milner derives from Blake's drawings some of the same points that we shall later derive from the Bible text.

It is possible to turn to Blake's drawings as a secondary but inexhaustible source of fresh ideas. For example, in the eleventh of the engravings which concerns the verses:

> Then thou scarest me with dreams, and terrifiest
> me through visions   (7: 14)

and

> My bones are pierced in me in the night season: and
> my sinews take no rest   (30: 17)

the sleeping figure of Job is in intimate contact with the godlike figure above and with other hands clasping him from below. This picture lends itself both to Freudian and Jungian interpretations of the content of unconscious processes. In Freudian terms, the dominant theme is the persecuting superego and Job could be seen to be in the centre of conflict. In Jungian terms, it would be necessary to look in the fine details for archetypal themes with contrary ideas. The God above is wrapped around by a serpent. The arm of the God above surrounds Job and also reaches one of the figures below who is tied in chains. Two other beings from below

---

[12] The word "wholeness" is more appropriate for this theme than the word "perfect" (see Chapter 2).

[13] Marion Milner, *op. cit.*, p. 32.

[14] *Ibid.*, p. 34.

appear to be holding on to the sleeping figure of Job. Job is thus an intermediary between the powers above and the powers below.

Jung has made a large number of references to the theme of Job, scattered throughout his collected works. In *Answer to Job*, he deals more comprehensively with the basic question for which Job demands an answer. We shall refer to some of these themes later.

MEDICAL INTERPRETATIONS

There are a number of references in which Job's illness is described in terms of categories of diseases in physical medicine. Most writers have thought of Job's illness in purely organic terms. Some have concentrated on the skin trouble (the boils) as a dermatological syndrome with, perhaps, the mental symptoms as secondary effects. Others have discussed the illness as being (amongst other suggestions) leprosy, pellagra, scurvy, and syphilis. There are two references to Job's illness as a psychosomatic condition (Guy and Halliday).

In 1887 Sir Risdon Bennett[15] concentrated on the physical aspect. He stated, concerning Job's running sores, that

> . . . whilst his physical condition was such as to previously impair his bodily health, his mental powers were retained. A very general belief has obtained that his disease was the true leprosy, the *elephantiasis Graecorum*.[16]

He added as another possibility, "that his malady may have been that peculiar Oriental sore known as the 'Aleppo or Bagdad evil'."[17]

A. Rendle-Short considers the likelihood of Job's illness being smallpox, but points out Dr. Orr-Ewing's thesis that Job probably suffered from a rare skin disease called dermatitis herpetiformis.[18]

An anonymous article by the librarian at the Army Medical Library of Washington, D.C.[19] gives abundant documentation to the tradition

---

[15] Sir Risdon Bennett, *The Diseases of the Bible* (Oxford: Horace Hart, 1887).

[16] *Ibid.*, p. 97.

[17] *Ibid.*, p. 100.

[18] A. Rendle-Short, *The Bible and Modern Medicine* (London: Paternoster Press, 1953), pp. 53–54.

[19] Librarian, Army Medical Library, "Morbus Jobi", *The Urologic and Cutaneous Review*, **40** (1936), pp. 296–299.

dating from the Middle Ages to the seventeenth century which saw Job's illness as syphilis. This traditional view is given credence by Job's reference to the punishment which he suffers at God's hands as the result of the iniquities of his youth (13: 26). Other diagnoses are mentioned, including Rollet's (1824–94) view that Job suffered from scurvy, although Buret (1891) pointed out that Job was too wealthy to have contracted this disease. Bousquillon (1802) thought that it was erysipelas, and Bloch (1901) believed it to be chronic eczema. This article concludes that there is not enough evidence in the text to support the view that Job suffered from any form of venereal disease, and that the "whole description is in general terms applicable to any ulcerative process".[20]

M. Webster Brown reports on the article of Dr. Trénel from *Paris Médical* which supports the claim that Job's illness was leprosy.[21]

Brim[22] is amongst those who came to the conclusion that Job's illness was due to a vitamin deficiency in the form of pellagra. Other writers have doubted this conclusion because they infer that, due to his wealth, Job would have been a well-fed man. Pellagra is a vitamin deficiency found amongst people who might live on agricultural lands but sell their produce for cash and live on cereals, being too poor to keep the more nutritious food for their own consumption. This pattern of living does not fit Job. However, pellagra is characterized by the "three Ds"—diarrhoea, dementia, and dermatitis, which were features of Job's affliction.

William Guy[23] refers to Job's illness as "psychosomatic". The dermatological condition

> appeared, lasted for a time, and then suddenly disappeared, just as do many cases of widespread lichen planus, psoriasis, atopic eczema, chronic urticaria, dermatitis herpetiformis, and generalized exfoliative dermatitis. The comings and goings of such dermatoses are enigmatic. We are as helpless in explaining them as were Job's ecclesiastical friends.[24]

---

[20] *Ibid.*, p. 299.

[21] M. Webster Brown, "Was Job a leper?", *Medical Journal and Record* (July 1933), pp. 32-33.

[22] Charles Brim, "Job's illness—pellagra", *Archives of Dermatology and Syphilology*, **46** (2) (Feb. 1942), pp. 371–376.

[23] William Guy, "Psychosomatic dermatology *circa* 400 B.C.", *Archives of Dermatology and Syphilology*, **71** (3) (March 1955), pp. 354–356.

[24] *Ibid.*, p. 356.

He goes on to say that

> The reasons for Job's physical sufferings are never explained. The mechanism of his recovery is obvious, but hard to put into present-day medical phraseology. Could you call it one more step in the process of maturation? Did his spiritual experience—his revelation of God—have a tranquilizing effect that healed him? Regardless, this profound and sophisticated work of religious literature should serve as a reminder to all physicians of psychosomatic bent that their thoughts have been pondered before, and long, long ago.[25]

The present work will centre upon the idea of the process of maturation, and we have found it interesting to note in searching the references that this idea had already been put forward in medical literature.

James Halliday[26] also discusses the psychosomatic aspect in Job's illness and considers that the Book of Job

> . . . enumerates a great variety of the bodily disturbances that follow upon an intensive emotional reaction to a disturbed life situation. From the psychiatric viewpoint of Jung it is worthy to remark that Job did not recover until he had come into contact with the archaic levels of the unconscious. After encountering in fantasy the phallic monsters of Behemoth and Leviathan and experiencing the whirlwind of the spirit his personality was, so to speak, reintegrated and concomitantly his somatic disorders resolved.[27]

We will discuss in a later chapter the unconscious aspect in its relation to the resolution of Job's illness.

It is the failing of the medical studies (with the exception of those of Guy and Halliday) that the skin disease is taken literally as being the illness. It is as if the smiting with sore boils was all that Job had to suffer. But to see the boils as the entire extent of Job's illness would deny validity to the course and outcome of the Biblical story and would regard his suffering as having no meaning beyond the physical complaints. If Job's illness is merely a fortuitous episode in a previously normal individual who became normal again as a result of his miraculous cure, then the meaning of the suffering as part of Job's development is lost. In our interpretation the illness is not seen as a transitory event with a cure as capricious as its onset. Our thesis is that Job's illness is part of a natural sequence in which

---

[25] William Guy, "Psychosomatic dermatology *cira* 400 B.C.", *Archives of Dermatology and Syphilology*, **71** (3) (March 1955), p. 356.

[26] James Halliday, "Psychosomatic medicine and the rheumatism problem", *The Practitioner*, **152** (Jan. 1944), pp. 6–15.

[27] *Ibid.*, p. 10.

the premorbid personality determines the particular kind of reaction of an individual to life's disasters. But the same features which provide the basis for morbid experiences are also able to be used creatively for the purpose of cure and further development.

Moreover, it is not so much that psychiatric knowledge will illuminate ideas about Job, but that the story of Job will illuminate the psychiatric approach to problems of mental illness. The aim is to relate the account of Job's life to three clinical syndromes which, although usually dealt with separately, can be shown to have connecting links in their psychopathology. The three syndromes are obsessional neurosis, depression, and paranoia. Extracts will be given from clinical descriptions from both traditional psychiatric sources and psychoanalytical writings. Events in Job's life, as delineated in the Bible account, will be related to these syndromes and to the underlying psychopathology. This will lead to speculation on the way in which mental illness impinges on human personality. In some cases it can be a disaster; in other cases it can be the stimulus to new levels of creative activity; more positively, it can result in a review of life aims, of ideas about God and the universe, and it can lead to new insights into the inner nature of man.

The story of Job is one of maturation to levels which could only be attained after intense inner suffering. The Bible story contains some basic ideas which are expressed in language which allows for a multiplicity of meanings. As stated earlier in this chapter, new meanings can be found in the Book of Job which have relevance to a contemporary scene far removed from the culture in which the ideas were first given shape. Each generation has the task of reconsidering the aims, purposes, and meanings of life in the idiom of its present, but borrowing from the accumulation of previous ideas embedded in the literature of the past.

This work should be seen as an attempt to reconsider some of the ideas expressed in the Book of Job. The idiom chosen is not exclusively a psychiatric one, but derives from it. It would have been impossible to work out these ideas without psychiatric experience. At the same time, it will be shown that the application of psychiatry to human problems can draw upon the literary and religious heritage in which the Book of Job has a unique place.

From a purely psychiatric point of view, it is possible to find in the Book of Job a sensitive and detailed account of the onset, course, and treatment of a mental disorder in which the most prominent feature is depression. There is an additional element: when the illness is resolved in the final chapters, a further stage is achieved—Job reaches a more mature level than that at which he had begun in his premorbid state. The vehicle by which his maturation is accomplished is, in fact, the very suffering which he undergoes.

The purpose of this book is to study the illness and the events surrounding it, and to find in the Bible story an account of some of the universal problems of mankind as revealed through critical events in the life of one individual. It is also concerned with the progression of ideas of human identity and the way in which human beings have searched for a harmony between experience of the self and experience of the universe.

CHAPTER 2

The Personality of Job
(The Premorbid Personality)

IN the previous chapter it was postulated that we were free to add new meanings to the Book of Job, and one might almost go so far as to say that it is obligatory on each generation to find its own special relevant message from the great literature that survives into it. The literature provides the living link between present and past, but it is always the present epoch which infuses life into that which the dead past has bequeathed.

Our initial theme depends upon meanings which can be attached to one single word used at the beginning of the Bible story to describe the personality of Job. The word is rendered variously in the English translations. In the Authorized and Revised Versions the word is rendered as "perfect"; in the translation by the American Jewish Publication Society (Soncino Books) it is rendered as "whole-hearted"; in the New English Bible Version it becomes "blameless".

The Hebrew word from which all these renderings are derived is *tam* (תָּם). The different meanings attached to the word *tam* provides us with our starting point to speculations about the nature of Job's personality in relation to his subsequent illness. Literally, *tam* means "whole" or "complete". In another context, that of selecting an animal for sacrifice (Exodus 12: 5 and Leviticus 5: 15), the same word is rendered as "without blemish". In that context it is intended to indicate that only an animal without physical flaw would be acceptable as a sacrifice to God. The idea of being without physical blemish also has an application to Job's original state of physical perfection in contrast with his subsequent affliction with boils. The first breach into his wholeness concerned his physical health.

In an abstract sense Job could be considered previously to have been without *moral* blemish.

A further elaboration of this latter meaning of wholeness can be found in the second chapter and subsequently, where reference is made to Job's "integrity",[1] which is the translation of the Hebrew word *tamat* (תמת), an abstract noun with the same root as the adjective *tam* appearing in the text as the compound word בתמתו. Working backwards from the word "integrity", the descriptions "perfect", "whole", "blameless", and "without blemish", could, in the modern psychological idiom, be rendered as "integrated". In this sense, we have a man whose personality was integrated and his illness is a breakdown of that integration (i.e. a disintegration of his personality).

Descriptions can carry value judgements, and the terms used to describe Job's personality reveal the degree of approval that would be given to the actions from which his reputation was gained. The words "whole", "complete", "whole-hearted", "without blemish", and "integrated" all carry approval such as that associated with the word "perfect", as used in both Authorized and Revised Versions of the Bible. Job's exemplary character represented the best in his own age, but, in our contemporary culture his "perfection" might not have been taken so readily for granted. The idea that he was an integrated personality could be challenged. The same behaviour which merited the description of "perfect" might well be described today as "perfectionist". This alteration would withdraw some of the approval. The word "conscientious" would retain more of the approval, but still would be less than perfect. If, however, we call Job's behaviour "obsessional", then we are taking it into the realms of pathology.

What is the evidence that gives us the right to assume these extensions of meaning with the Bible text?

First, when Job is described as leading a "blameless and upright life", he is considered to be doing so in so far as he "feared God and set his face against wrongdoing" (1: 2). Marion Milner aptly comments on this text:

> Thus he is shown persistently denying that there could be any evil in himself; and he is shown as able to do this because he believes only in the conscious life,

---

[1] God says to Satan, "You incited me to ruin him without a cause, but his integrity is still unshaken" (2: 3). Job's wife says to him, "Are you still unshaken in your integrity?" (2: 9).

he believes that because his conscious intention is good and solely devoted to the worship and service of God, therefore he must be good.[2]

Job's insistence on what has been called his perfection—the lack of any flaw in his character—is a trait seen in obsessional personalities.

Moreover, we find that he is over-concerned about his seven sons and three daughters. His children were accustomed to feasting in turn, "each one upon his day", and it occurred to Job to sacrifice not only on his own account, but on their behalf as well, "for he thought that they might somehow have sinned against God and committed blasphemy in their hearts. *This he always did*" (1:15).[3] Job is not aware of any sins of his own, nor indeed of any sins of his children, but he takes responsibility for their religious observance and their morality. Job, in fact, denies his children a separate identity in that he takes upon himself the responsibility for making sacrifices on their behalf, and for absolving them from sins which they *might* have committed.

Many psychiatric case histories include details of rituals which people undertake in order to avert personal disaster or to avoid such a fate falling upon a member of the family. Any failure to carry out the ritual would result in misfortune. It is as if this person were saying, "My omissions are my own and their omissions are mine also, because I know better; and, for that reason, I carry more responsibility than they do." Job's religious activities were performed ostensibly to safeguard the fate of his children. They could just as well have been performed in order to safeguard his own peace of mind, for his sons and daughters, included amongst his possessions, are part of his sense of identity. The text confirms this view:

> He had seven sons and three daughters; and he owned seven thousand sheep and three thousand camels, five hundred yoke of oxen and five hundred asses, with a large number of slaves. *Thus*[4] Job was the greatest man in all the East.
> (1: 2–3)

Possessions contribute to the image of the self, and when the possessions include family members, obsessional processes may be used in order to preserve their lives and control their fate. The obsessional activity provides a safeguard for the well-being of those who figure closely in the obsessional individual's life.

[2] Marion Milner, *op. cit.*, p. 31.
[3] Our italics.
[4] Our italics.

Job's greatness and his perfection are thus connected with his possessions and the lives of his children. The breakdown of his physical and mental integration is associated with the loss of his children and his wealth. Far from being perfect, Job's personality contained features which in our own culture might be considered to be the precursor of mental breakdown.

The idea of Job's perfection has been so far considered as appertaining to his premorbid personality. This character trait became submerged during the illness, and yet something of it survived through the period of his abasement to re-emerge in his final survey of his case. The whole of chapter 29 is a reassertion of his perfection. He refers to "the old days" and gives details of the general acceptance of his greatness (29: 7–25). Job continues to list his virtues, describing his good deeds on behalf of the poor man, the orphan, the widow, the blind, the lame, and the needy. In all this, "I put on righteousness as a garment and it clothed me" (29: 14).

In this passage, however, there is a sentence which is relevant to the nature of his illness and the cure in which we wish to anticipate some of the themes of our later chapters:

> I thought, "I shall die with my powers unimpaired
> and my days uncounted as the grains of sand,
> with my roots spreading out to the water
> and the dew lying on my branches,
> with the bow always new in my grasp
> and the arrow ever ready to my hand."
>
> (29: 18–20)

Here one can picture the man whose strength is part of his personal identity. Any erosion of that strength threatens the total image of the self. This is not an unfamiliar characteristic of men who are authoritarian in their own families and leaders in the community, and who would prefer to die in harness than to experience a diminution of their powers. There are those who die within weeks of their retirement, and those who become ill in anticipation of a challenge from a younger man.

Every culture has its normalities and abnormalities, and it might be expected that the explanations for any breakdown of personality would embody, amongst other factors, the values of the period of time, geographical area, social class, and prevailing religious beliefs. Even within one culture, a particular piece of behaviour can be given descriptions on a

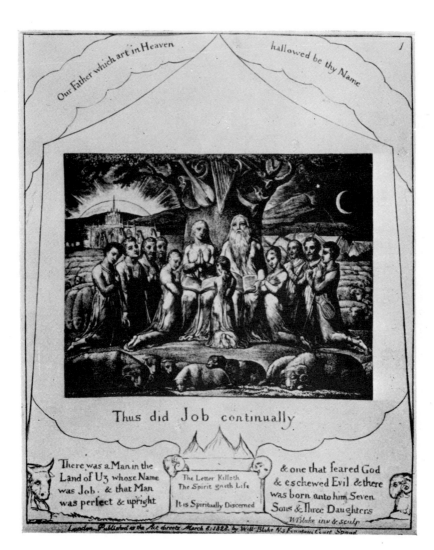

Our Father which art in Heaven   hallowed be thy Name

Thus did Job continually

The Letter Killeth
The Spirit giveth Life

It is Spiritually Discerned

There was a Man in the
Land of Uz whose Name
was Job. & that Man
was perfect & upright

& one that feared God
& eschewed Evil & there
was born unto him Seven
Sons & Three Daughters

W Blake inv & sculp

London. Published as the Act directs March 8: 1825. by Will Blake N 3 Fountain Court Strand

hierarchy of esteem which depends upon the usefulness of the results. We may distinguish between obsessional personality, which is a description of variations within the normal, and obsessional neurosis, which is the name of a mental disorder. An individual with obsessional personality traits may find fulfilment in occupations which require an exact and conscientious approach, and it would be inappropriate to use derogatory or pathological labels in describing him. The same qualities, however, could be a hindrance in any occupation and personal relationships which depend upon recognizing broad principles, and where it is necessary to tolerate ambiguity of meanings in a single phrase, or the possibility of alternative choices of equal value in the approach to a problem. The obsessional personality works well when an answer to a problem with which he is confronted is right or wrong, according to accepted standards. Where the result of some act cannot be anticipated, or where known standards do not apply, the obsessional personality finds the doubt intolerable. There is no room in this type of personality for approximate justice in relation to behaviour or approximate rewards for services rendered. He is not capable of taking part in the happy give-and-take of many ordinary relationships. The obsessional personality also finds it difficult to adapt to alterations in techniques and attitudes in a changing world.

So long as the obsessional features seem to be congruous with the individual's self-image, and so long as they find useful outlets, they are merely part of the ordinary differences between people. Nevertheless, an obsessional personality is a vulnerable personality. There is a point at which the obsessional features can become too heavy a burden. This is where the boundary between normality and abnormality is crossed. The individual no longer finds himself at an advantage in some areas of living, and has to acknowledge an inner compulsion which is no longer compatible with his idea of his own personality. This is the point at which one refers to the condition of "obsessional neurosis".

There are some psychiatric writers who would distinguish clearly obsessional neurosis, which is an illness, from obsessional personality, which is a variant of the normal. Psychoanalytical writers refer not only to the *illness* and the *personality* but to the *obsessional process* which pervades human beings to different degrees at different phases of their lives. The obsessional process can be related historically in an individual's life to the stages in his psychosexual development. This forms part of the contribution of psychoanalytical ideas to the understanding of some of the disturbing features of ordinary life.

Obsessional processes as a morbid feature have been described revealingly by Wilhelm Stekel. Emil Gutheil, who translated Stekel's *Compulsion and Doubt*, contributes an introduction to the book in which there are ideas which are relevant to the theme of Job. He lists amongst obsessional symptomatology the ceremonialism in everyday life. Fear of the emptiness of life is a prime motive for the patient to give himself up to endless repetitions:

> Most compulsion neurotics . . . ascribe good or bad omens to many trivial actions. In the patient's mind, trifles receive mystical value, while great and important experiences are underestimated.[5]

This refers to transactions between man and God or the Supernatural, but it applies equally to transactions and arguments with fellow men. The obsessional person may be completely unable to see and deal with the main point at issue, but he can usually succeed in argument because he is so prolific in meticulously observed detail. There is always another trivial side issue at hand which he can use to evade the discussion of the essence of the topic.

This hypersensitivity to detail can lead to what Gutheil calls a *manie de perfection*:

> Whatever the patient does must be done in a perfect manner: washing, counting' walking, praying, thinking. . . . No truly religious person is so careful to collect such intense concentration and devotion for his prayer as the compulsion neurotic does. Imperfection is a natural quality of the mortal, a law a compulsion neurotic refuses to accept. But the patient is troubled with doubts, and his desire for perfection propels him to an endless repetition compulsion.[6]

By relying on his perfection, the patient feels himself to be in the right on any question which may arise in daily living. He only admits disease when the expectancies which he has are obviously not met by his real-life situation: when fate, in a sense, lets him down.

[5] Wilhelm Stekel, *Compulsion and Doubt*, trans. Emil A. Gutheil (New York: Liveright Publishing Corp., 1949), p. 9.

[6] *Ibid.*, pp. 9–10.

Thus, it is possible to infer from the text that Job endeavoured to maintain his position and definition of himself as the greatest man in the East by his ritual observances on behalf of his children. His observances assured his good fortune and theirs. By taking over the responsibility for his childrens' moral behaviour, he hoped to maintain a state of grace for them which would avert any disaster that might befall them and, by inference, avoid what such a disaster would mean to his own definition of himself as "blameless and upright".

In spite of his rituals, bad fortune does befall him. He loses children and possessions. *The bad fortune is also the loss of the good fortune that he feels entitled to.* His belief that he possessed control over his fate and his self-definition was demolished. A further loss was his belief that his rituals and his "perfect" behaviour controlled God.

Gutheil points out that among the mechanisms of obsessional neurosis, the unintelligible words or fragments of sentences are repetitiously thought or spoken out loud. These are "products of condensation, similar to those found in dreams".[7] They are the results of reasonings which have a meaning for the patient but which are unintelligible when they arise in the flow of normal conversation. This can be related to the tangential nature of the cycles of speeches and responses which occur between Job and the comforters. Job's repetitious use of legal terminology and argumentation, for example, find no response from the comforters. They in turn dwell on repentance in the face of what they assume to be God's meting out of justice for past sins committed either by Job or his children. This is an idea of divine justice which Job is able to refute within his own terms of reference. The comforters not only do not acknowledge his terms, they also make no response to his words.

Another mechanism which occurs in obsessional neurosis is an attempt to eliminate death. The obsession becomes the means by which the patient remains in a netherland beyond the laws of life and death.

> The rare moments in which he perceives the passing of time are intolerable to him. His time is spent on ceremonials, systems, fantasies and doubts, and on checking and rechecking his pseudo-activities. He may also act similarly toward sleep. . . . He may postpone the hours of sleep and in this symbolic fashion postpone the hour of his death.[8]

---

[7] *Ibid.*, p. 11.
[8] *Ibid.*, p. 14.

Even though Job had claimed at certain depressive stages that he wishes death to blacken out his suffering, he describes how difficult it is for him to sleep and the fact that he can find no comfort in sleep:

> troubled nights are my lot.
> When I lie down, I think,
> "When will it be day that I may rise?"
> When the evening grows long and I lie down
> I do nothing but toss till morning twilight.
>
> (7: 3–4)

In another passage, Job contemplates death and the possibility of suicide, and realizes that his religiosity will make no difference to him in the grave:

> If I measure Sheol for my house,
> if I spread my couch in the darkness,
> if I call the grave my father
> and the worm my mother or my sister,
> where, then, will my hope be,
> and who will take account of my piety?
> I cannot take them down to Sheol with me,
> nor can they descend with me into the earth.
>
> (17: 13–16)

The comfort which he derives from his piety will not go with him to the grave. There he would be bereft of the sustaining qualities that come from his obsessional traits and would have to face his being-in-death, in a sense, naked. And yet in another sense this passage implies that he is making friends with death and thereby making death the equivalent of another existence.

Gutheil considers the obsessional mechanisms which have to do with truth and falsehood (secrets) and good and bad behaviour (moral and immoral imperatives). Underlying the obsession is an active feeling of guilt which the obsession attempts to hide. The guilt is present but not recognized consciously, and there is an endeavour to avoid coming to terms with the unconscious guilt by insisting on overzealous concern for the absolute truth, sincerity, and uprightness. This extreme concern for the "truth" betrays the fear of a concealed truth behind the compulsions. An examination of the patient's inner motives would reveal criminal tendencies for which the compulsions are outward compensations. A compulsion neurosis "offers the patient protection against his own anti-social impulses".[9] Job himself gives what might be a description of a compulsive activity which results in keeping him free from the feeling of sinfulness:

> I stitched sackcloth together to cover my body
> and I buried my forelock in the dust;
> my cheeks were flushed with weeping
> and dark shadows were round my eyes,
> yet my hands were free from violence
> and my prayer was sincere.   (16: 15–17)

If religion is one sign of a developed civilization where moral laws are established on behalf of society in an attempt to keep primitive impulses in check, then the rituals of compulsion, which Freud called a "private religion", are attempts by the obsessional individual to protect himself and those around him from the consequences of his unconscious rebellion against the established codes:

> In accordance with the primitive level of the patient's personality his rituals are very cruel, requiring utmost self-sacrifice and self-humiliation, and depriving him of all personal happiness. . . . Most patients of this type . . . are candidates for suicide, but lack the courage to commit suicide; just as they are criminals without the courage to commit a crime.[10]

These patients go to great lengths to prove that they do not harbour the very criminal impulses which they unconsciously wish to indulge:

> We often find compulsion neurotics apprehensive lest they be taken for swindlers. The reaction formations are hyper-correctness and hyper-conscientiousness. Their doubt is justified to a certain degree because they are constantly exposed to a pressure of unconscious criminal wishes.[11]

These people are meticulously honest because they sense that their unlawful tendencies might be easily exposed. It is relevant here to point out the extent to which Job insisted on his righteous behaviour and his complete lack of sinfulness. Over and over again he asserts his claim to perfection and even goes so far as to enumerate all the sins he had *not* committed:

[9] *Ibid.*, p. 19.
[10] *Ibid.*, p. 18.
[11] *Ibid.*, p. 19.

> I put on righteousness as a garment and it clothed me;
> justice, like a cloak or a turban, wrapped me round.
> I was eyes to the blind
> and feet to the lame;
> I was a father to the needy,
> and I took up the stranger's cause.
>
> (29: 14–16)

He emphasizes his generosity and benevolence:

> If I have withheld their needs from the poor
> or let the widow's eye grow dim with tears,
> if I have eaten my crust alone,
> and the orphan has not shared it with me—
> . . .
> then may my shoulder-blade be torn from my shoulder,
> my arm be wrenched out of its socket!   (31: 16–22)

Indeed, the whole of chapter 31 of the Bible story is devoted to Job's enumeration and illustration of the fact that he did not break any one of the Mosaic laws.

Gutheil concludes with a description of the major difference between paranoid states, depression, and obsessional neurosis:

> In paranoid conditions the patient is convinced that the world is responsible for his suffering. In melancholic conditions the patient feels himself responsible for the suffering of the whole world. In compulsion diseases, however, the patient must sacrifice his own happiness in order to save the world from suffering.[12]

The fact that these three conditions—obsessional neurosis, depression, and paranoia—are different expressions of the same morbidity is a major theme of this work. It is important to note at this stage that Gutheil relates all three to the question of suffering and responsibility, and points out that in compulsion neurosis the moral imperative is a prime element. He states that:

> In this "private religion" (Freud) all questions of the civilized man, "May I?" "Can I?" "Shall I?" are answered with a categorical "You must!" And yet underlying doubts dispel much of the strength of this categorical imperative. The patient must repeat his actions again and again, and it is as though some of

---

[12] Wilhelm Stekel, *Compulsion and Doubt*, p. 24.

the eternal questions of civilization were asked, and were to be answered, again and again.[13]

As we have already noted, Job was accustomed to performing over and over again the same religious sacrifices on behalf of his children, "for he thought that they might somehow have sinned against God and committed blasphemy in their hearts. This he always did" (1: 15). At this stage Job may be a slave to the compulsive element behind his actions, but he would not wish what he feels to be his "principles" to be any different.

His breakdown occurs when the burden of maintaining the rectitude behind his actions becomes too great for his resources. In the breakdown of the obsessional personality, an individual may pass quickly through obsessional neurosis into a depressive state.

We can now examine some of the symptoms which Job describes. They are the evidence of the breakdown of his personality, and they follow a course which extends through the different stages of his illness and become resolved at the point of his final recovery.

[13] *Ibid.*, pp. 18–19.

CHAPTER 3

The Symptoms of
Job's Illness

FOR the purpose of this chapter, the Bible text will be considered as recording the words of a living person, and we shall look upon these words as being Job's own communications about his feelings and experiences.

It is not our chosen task to comment on the poetic quality of Job's speeches. The language is appropriate to the intensity of the emotion which is being experienced. It is our purpose to draw conclusions about these experiences using the kind of reasoning which would be available to a clinician who was faced with communications of this nature. The words themselves provide material which the clinician uses in attempting to understand the distress of those who seek his aid. Although the clinical framework is not the only one within which people communicate about their disturbances, it is being used here in order to provide a modern perspective of age-old problems. This allows us to deal with Job's experiences and feelings as being the equivalent of symptoms of illness.

Job describes his sufferings in great detail. All that he expresses about his experience of what he has lost stands out in contrast with his experience of initial perfection. The story has become a paradigm of the effects of disaster on the personality of an individual.

In Job's case there was a man of consistent good fortune and good health who loses both in quick succession. The ordinary course of human existence, however, is a series of changes and adaptations, a large number of which are inherent in the biological processes of development, and others which form part of each individual's fair share of the chance events which human beings encounter in the material and social environment with which they interact. Even the changes which are points of progress can become critical stages of adaptation at which disturbances may arise. Human development is concerned with the facts of life, which include birth, death, illness, satisfactions, privations, growth, decay, renewal, regression, interaction, isolation. Experiences may be described as good or bad, and, on another scale of values, as healthy or ill. The ordinary individual experiences a changing balance of goodness and badness, and health and illness. What we ordinarily describe as health and good fortune is the balance which is satisfactory enough for the time being, and which is subject to change—sometimes in the direction of improvement and at others of worsening. There is a view of human development which finds a value for every stage of life, from infancy to old age. But it has always been difficult to find a satisfactory explanation for unanticipated calamities, illnesses, and early death.

Mental illness is a case in point. The questions, how and why do the symptoms occur, are fundamental issues in the study of human nature. No final answer is to be expected. The value of any theoretical study of symptom formation is judged by the usefulness of the results in practice.

The process of psychogenic symptom formation has been considered in three separate dimensions. The first is that of *critical periods* in the life cycle in which emotional hazards may occur. Within this dimension symptom formation is related to immediate situations. Symptoms arise when the adaptation to these situations is faulty in some way. The second dimension is the *psychodynamic* one, in which psychopathology in adults is traced to earlier experiences in childhood and infancy. The third dimension is the *cultural* one, in which personal reactions are seen in relation to the repertoires of behaviour which are available in any particular culture.

Crisis theory, which relates to the stages in the life cycle which contain emotional hazards, was originally developed by Lindemann,[1] and the concept was later elaborated by Caplan[2] in order to provide a basis for helpful intervention at points of stress. In crisis theory there is concentration

---

[1] E. Lindemann, "Symptomatology and management of acute grief", *Am. J. Psychiat.* **101** (1944).

[2] G. Caplan, *Concepts of Mental Health Consultation* (Children's Bureau, U.S. Dept. of H.E.W., Washington D.C., U.S.A. Publication No. 373, 1959).

on a series of events in the life of an individual and on the way that adaptation is made to them. On the psychodynamic level there is concentration on the personal history of the individual as related to the development of the inner psychic processes. In the cultural dimension there is emphasis on the standards of value in the community and on individual adjustment to them.

Many clinicians have enclosed themselves within a single one of these three systems. These are the people who, by their exclusive attention to one level, have extended the area of work within that dimension. But we shall find in referring to the story of Job that any or all of these dimensions may be applicable at different stages, and, on some occasions, all three levels are operative at the same time.

At the level of crisis theory, Job's illness could be considered as a reaction to the calamities which befell him. These calamities differed only by their intensity from events which would be familiar to his contemporaries. Every individual is subject to hazards. Family life is an interweaving of sorrows and joys. Illnesses, deaths, losses of fortune or of esteem run parallel with births, marriages, success, and personal growth. The Job story concentrates on events subsequent to the greatest conceivable loss, and on the manner of his adaptation to it.

Crisis theory also takes into account both the outcome of previous crises (which makes the individual either more vulnerable or more resistant to subsequent stresses) and the kind of support which is available in the immediate situation. An enduring pattern of reaction is built up over a series of crises.

At the moment of crisis the individual is subject to stresses which may come from the outside, but the occasion provides an opportunity for change which comes from within. This is the creative potential of the crisis which allows the attainment of levels of development which had not previously been achieved. The movement towards mental health or mental ill health depends largely on the kind of interaction which takes place between the individual and key figures in his social environment. The implication for psychiatric services is that intervention in a crisis is not exclusively an activity for professional psychiatric personnel, but that help can by given by a variety of semi-professional and non-professional helpers—relatives, friends, neighbours, and members of the community: the supporters and helpers.

The next level at which symptom formation can be considered represents the psychodynamic schools of psychological medicine. Each illness has its separate psychopathology. Precipitating events are taken into account only in relation to the psychic processes which are the resultant of all the mental events in the course of the individual's development. Here, too, there is more than one way in which the dimension can be explored, but the emphasis is on the personal content of the individual's mental processes and on the way that he perceives the outside world. Notwithstanding the effect of immediate precipitating events, adult pathology is thought to have its roots in infancy. Symptoms are the result of defences against conflicts which include unconscious as well as conscious features.

The third level, the cultural one, is the one which has been explored more by modern sociologists than by clinicians. Mental illness is described as a social role imposed upon the individual by others. Human beings arrange themselves in categories of esteem and place some people at a disadvantage by applying stigma to kinds of behaviour which at one particular moment attract popular disapproval. In this dimension mental illness is "deviancy" by popular consent. This view has been put forward by Szasz,[3] and by Laing who states that "sanity or psychosis is tested by the degree of conjunction or disjunction between two persons where the one is sane by common consent".[4] This dimension, in a more general way, allows for the recognition of the fact that mental illness is relative to the culture, and that ideas about mental illness can alter. It may be possible at times to find value in mental disorder by looking upon it as a rebellion against outworn cultural values.

These three dimensions (critical situations, individual psychopathology, cultural maladaptation) refer to the way in which symptoms come into being. We need another framework in which to organize the description of the varying nature of the symptoms themselves. Psychiatry depends upon diagnosis which goes further than deciding whether a person is mentally disordered or not. It is the discovery of regularly occurring patterns in mental disorder, and each pattern forms a distinctive diagnostic category.

[3] T. Szasz, "The myth of mental illness", in T. Scheff (Ed.), *Mental Illness and Social Processes*, (New York: Harper & Row, 1967).
[4] R. D. Laing, *The Divided Self* (London: Tavistock Publications, 1960), p. 37.

Out of the large number of diagnostic categories and sub-categories which have been built up in psychiatric practice in order to record and compare observations on the nature and treatment of mental disorder, we shall select three broad groups as being relevant to our consideration of the description of Job's experiences: *psychosomatic disease, psychoneurosis*, and *psychosis*.

We are avoiding all the detailed categories used nationally and internationally. Even those who pay the greatest attention to the specific nature of psychiatric syndromes have to acknowledge the fact that these syndromes are an artificial creation for the purpose of classification. Aubrey Lewis, calling attention to the difficulty of identifying clinical syndromes as separate specific entities, states that:

> . . . there is an undoubtedly large, if unnumbered, part of the population who have mild mental disorder not needing mental hospital care: hysteria, obsessional neurosis, hypochondria, chronic depression, paranoid states, and so forth. The diversity of this widespread group of illnesses depends on their being disorders of mind—disorders, that is, of the human function which comprehends and sums up all other functions of the organism, serves to relate a human being to his complex environment, and is the chief token that he is an individual, and not a sample. Mental disorders are therefore varied, as are the people who suffer from them. It is only by ignoring most of what is individual in these illnesses that a few common types or categories can be recognised, comparable to the "diseases" of somatic medicine. Such a procedure is necessary for practical ends; material must be classified.[5]

We have chosen our broad categories as representing a gradation in complexity of reaction. In *psychosomatic disorders* the body speaks for the disturbance of mind; the *psychoneuroses* are mainly psychic experiences; and in the *psychoses* the total personality of the individual is involved.

A psychosomatic illness is a general psychic disturbance with local organic symptoms. The symptoms are transformations of psychic stress and conflict into bodily dysfunction. Glover points out that the difference between these symptoms and those of psychoneuroses lies in their respective etiology:

> . . . it is possible to draw two fundamental distinctions between the psycho-neuroses and all psycho-somatic disorders, first, that the process of symptom-formation in the psycho-neuroses follows a standardized psychic pattern and

---

[5] Aubrey Lewis, "Psychological medicine", in F. W. Price (Ed.), *A Textbook of the Practice of Medicine* (London: Oxford University Press, 1947), p. 1835.

second, that the psycho-neuroses have psychic content and meaning. Psycho-somatic disorders on the other hand, although influenced by psychic reactions at some point or another in their progress, have in themselves no psychic content, and consequently do not present stereotyped patterns of conflict.[6]

Glover considers that a traumatic factor or an anxiety factor is often fundamental to psychosomatic disorders. An example would be the sudden loss of a family member which causes depression with guilt features:

> . . . the fusion of grief, anxiety, guilt and hate present in organised depression interferes radically with the free discharge of instinct excitations. Hence the common attribution of certain gastro-intestinal "organ neuroses" to undis-charged grief.[7]

Such symptoms arise when the ego is no longer able to master tension or to discharge it normally,[8] and converts the resultant psychic energy into bodily disorders. Matching symptom to symptom and experience to experience, it will be noted that Glover's observations correspond closely with details of Job's complaints as described in the Bible text. Glover also lists dermatoses, respiratory disorders, constipation or diarrhoea, sleep disorders, and muscular malfunctions (tremblings and tics).[9]

When we come to the description of Job's obsessional activities, we pass into the category of psychoneurosis. But the obsessional states are charac-teristically in the borderland between mental disorder and the psycho-pathology of everyday life. *These obsessional processes are also the link between the personal pathology and the cultural factors.*

In Job's case, our evidence for the obsessional processes is in his sacri-fices on behalf of his children, *lest* they had sinned, and in his insistence throughout the Bible narrative on his "perfect" behaviour. This extension of responsibility is often concurrent with ambivalent feelings towards the object for which responsibility is felt. In a patriarchal family system, close family members, especially offspring, might well be considered as poten-tial threats to the authority of the father. This threat may be a factor which the conscious facility is unable to recognize, because the threat would elicit

[6] Edward Glover, *Psycho-Analysis* (London: Staples Press, 1949), pp. 170–171.

[7] *Ibid.*, p. 174.

[8] *Ibid.*, p. 172.

[9] During the course of the Bible story, Job will experience many of these symp-toms.

a desire to eliminate the source of danger. Job's over-solicitude for the moral safety of his children could have been the counterpart of his wish to harm them. His sacrifices, which were intended for their benefit in relation to God, may also have been undertaken in an effort to avoid the effects of the hostile component of his own ambivalent feelings.

The various syndromes of psychoneuroses differ in the intensity of the reaction to an inner conflict and/or an external stress. The first stage in the response to stress is the release of chemical substances which produce physiological changes and a psychic experience of unease. This is the basis of anxiety, which is a psychophysical state. In small doses, anxiety serves the purpose of mobilizing the individual's resources to meet a challenge. Excessive doses of anxiety paralyze the individual's capacity to cope with external sources of stress. The undischarged anxiety becomes a new source of danger from within, and elaborate systems of physical and mental defences are then built up. This is the beginning of symptom formation.

Illness, for all its dangers and discomforts, brings some privileges, or primary gains, which attach to the status of the sick person. The gains and losses are somewhat capricious; the defences sometimes fail; and the primary gain may become lost in the discomfort, distress, and the loss of function which the symptoms bring about.

There are many categories within the psychoneuroses. The syndromes that are particularly relevant to Job are the *obsessional* and *phobic* states.

Phobias, which are irrational fears of objects, people, or situations, are a psychic representation of anxiety which threatens the personality from within, without any identifiable external source. Fears of dirt, darkness, illness, death, as well as claustrophobic fears,[10] are all factors which can be seen as threats distintegrating to the psyche. The function of phobia formation lies in

> increasing the *psychic distance* between the unconscious source of fear and its expression in fear of a consciously recognized situation or object.[11]

---

[10] At one time or another, Job expresses all of these fears. It suffices to quote at this point his description of how he feels that God has hemmed him in:

> He has walled in my path so that I cannot break away,
> and he has hedged in the road before me.   (19 : 8)

[11] Edward Glover, *op. cit.*, p. 153.

Obsessions are attempts to ward off dangers by compulsive repetitions of thoughts, words, and/or deeds. The function of obsessional symptom formation differs from that of phobic processes in so far as the latter project immediate representations of danger onto the psyche, whereas the former constitute attempts by the psyche to avoid, divert, or obliviate the sources of danger. The threat actually lies in the individual's own unrecognized ambivalent feelings towards a real object in his life.

This element of ambivalence necessitates the repression of the dangerous impulses. The compulsive activities form a kind of screen between conscious intentions and unconscious impulses. The good activity conceals the bad thoughts.

A resultant element in obsessional symptom formation is that of doubt and uncertainty. It is as if the doubt were better than the certainty of disaster which would be the consequence of the unconscious hate feelings. Freud revealed the occurrence of doubt in obsessional symptoms:

> The predilection felt by obsessional neurotics for uncertainty and doubt leads them to turn their thoughts by preference to those subjects upon which all mankind are uncertain and upon which our knowledge and judgements must necessarily remain open to doubt. The chief subjects of this kind are paternity, length of life, life after death, and memory. . . .[12]

Throughout the speeches, Job repeatedly explores those areas of human concern which enter into the realms of philosophical and religious inquiry. His questioning of the accepted religious viewpoints of his day bring him to new levels of understanding that go beyond the traditional norms that are given expression by the comforters. On one level, his doubting of accepted standards, and of the traditional answers to the basic questions of the human situation, is consistent with the symptoms of obsessional states. On another level, his doubts on matters which were taken for certainties in his time (especially those concerning divine justice) opened him up to a kind of experience which stretches the human imagination, and which is included amongst the most creative of human endeavours. It is in this sense that we can speak of Job as experiencing a creative illness.

[12] Sigmund Freud, "A case of obsessional neurosis" (1909), *Standard Edition*, Vol. X (London: Hogarth Press, 1955), p. 232.

The third level of syndrome is that of the psychoses, and here we have the greatest semantic problem. If we recognize a psychotic process in an individual, we have to acknowledge that it does not necessarily commit us to labelling him as insane. There is a borderland of sanity and insanity into which every individual enters, even if only in his dreams. The ordinary individual experiences in some degree, and at some moments of his life, every symptom which forms part of the illness in the most severe mental disorders. Thus it can be said that psychosis is not completely alien to the sane individual. But beyond this shared experience, there are points on the scale of sanity and insanity at which the balance seems to be tilted towards psychosis. An individual who is at one of these points may still maintain some links with his own sanity, and with some greater or lesser fragment of the world in which he is living. The point that we wish to make is that Job entered into psychotic processes which are clearly recognizable as being of the very same nature as those in mentally ill patients who suffer (in particular) from *depression*, which is part of the manic-depressive process, and *paranoia*, which is part of a schizophrenic process. Those two particular processes of a psychotic nature are indicated in the very descriptions Job uses about his feelings and experiences.

Freud entered into the semantic issue when distinguishing the nature of melancholia from mourning. He took grief, which is a normal experience, and contrasted it with depression, which is pathology, finding features in common and areas of differences. This is where the single clinical syndrome is seen to be most inappropriate as an exclusive explanation. When labels like "depression" and "paranoia" are used without qualification, it is possible to miss the fact that the normal person is familiar with such experiences. These experiences become mental illness as much by their intensity as by their quality.

Clinical studies give ample evidence of the fact that, in the depression which follows loss, where grief is present, anger is not far away. In some senses, the clinical state of depression differs from the normal experience of mourning in that the anger is turned inwards on the individual's own physical and mental processes. Freud stated that:

> The distinguishing mental features of melancholia are a profoundly painful dejection, abrogation of interest in the outside world, loss of the capacity to love, inhibition of all activity, and a lowering of the self-regarding feelings to a degree that finds utterance in self-reproaches and self-revilings, and culminates in

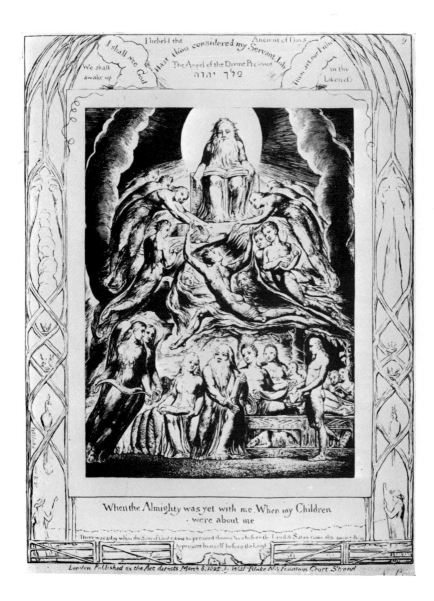

When the Almighty was yet with me. When my Children
were about me

a delusional expectation of punishment. This picture becomes a little more intel-
ligible when we consider that, with one exception, the same traits are met with
in grief. The fall in self-esteem is absent in grief; but otherwise the features are
the same.[13]

Freud came to the conclusion that "the loss of the object became transformed into a loss in the ego".[14] The loss becomes a threat to the sense of
identity.

In descriptions within clinical psychiatry, paranoia and depression are
clearly distinguished from one another. And yet in both cases the apparent
precipitating factor is the experience of some loss.

The essential feature in the clinical criteria for the diagnosis of paranoia
is that the individual experiences feelings of persecution that are a fantasy.
But the paranoid process has been studied by sociologists for the good
reason that the perception of actual or threatened loss may have some
basis in reality. Moreover, the paranoid person may well have suffered
from recognizable attempts to exclude him from his family or occupational
group, and precipitating events of the disorder may include actual experiences of discrimination. Paranoia is therefore part of an interaction with
other people and not a condition which is enclosed within one individual.
The situation is well described by Lemert:

> The paranoid process begins with some actual or threatened loss of status for the
> individual. This is related to such things as the death of relatives, failure to be
> promoted, age and physiological life cycle changes, mutilations, and change in
> family and marital relationships. The status changes are distinguished by the
> fact that they leave no alternative acceptable to the individual, from whence
> comes their "intolerable" or "unendurable" quality.[15]

It would seem that, whereas in some cases the experience of loss initiates
depression, in another individual an almost exactly similar experience is
the apparent starting point of the paranoid process.

Melanie Klein formulated a comprehensive system of developmental
psychology which shows the connections between paranoia and depression. In the earliest stages of infant development the boundaries of the

[13] Sigmund Freud, "Mourning and melancholia" (1917), *Standard Edition*, Vol.
XIV (London: Hogarth Press, 1957), p. 244.
[14] *Ibid.*, p. 159.
[15] E. M. Lemert, "Paranoia and the dynamics of exclusion", in T. J. Scheff (Ed.),
Mental Illness and Social Processes (New York: Harper & Row, 1967), p. 278.

"self" are blurred. The experience of goodness and badness, whether coming from inside or from outside, has no clear location. Feelings of anger or discomfort as experienced within the self are indistinguishable from external attacks, whereas comfort and satisfaction are felt as the goodness of the whole universe. This is a magical world in which it is possible to influence and be influenced by other people, and where inner thoughts and feelings can be destructive to another person's existence. This is the "paranoid position" as described by Melanie Klein, and the processes in this phase may be preserved and reactivated in the adult.

The "depressive position" is the result of some degree of integration of the personality. The body image is more clearly defined. Using the metaphor of good objects and bad objects, which are introjected from external sources, it is possible to recognize satisfaction and discomfort as being located in the self. Goodness and badness likewise can be perceived as existing in the single figure of the nurturing adult. There is no need to separate the world into clear categories of uniform goodness and badness. At this stage the infant has sufficient integration to experience the reality of the loss of something that is good, and to acknowledge the reality of a harmful experience. The experience of simultaneous goodness and badness is part of the ambivalence of interpersonal relationships.

The adult who is depressed is distraught because he may equate the hostile component of his ambivalent feelings with the cause of some person's death. At the same time, the loss of that person is the loss of a possession (an internal object). In the paranoid adult, any such internal loss is felt to be the equivalent of an attack coming from the outside.

The paranoid position and the depressive position are in the first place related to chronological stages of normal development, but the concept has an additional importance in that the same processes may be reactivated in successive stages during the life span. Some of the earliest experiences of loss may set the pattern for the type of reaction to subsequent events. Thus the outer manifestation of the experience of loss depends upon the stage at which the first loss is felt.

Our task is now to link these present-day descriptions of clinical syndromes and mental processes with the Bible descriptions of the personality of Job. We do not wish to force our interpretation of the Job story into the pattern of any one theory of symptom formation, nor compress the description of his illness into any one clinical syndrome. To do so would do an injustice to the magnitude of Job's experience and would reduce the number of meanings which can be applied to the descriptions. The descriptions nevertheless carry clear allusions to feelings, thoughts, and behaviour which, in a modern setting, would be termed symptoms of a mental disorder.

The demonstration of this relationship has its difficulties, and among the most important of these is the problem of distinguishing a "personality feature", which an individual feels to be an essential part of his personality, from a "symptom", which he feels has come upon him unaccountably. We must scrutinize the Bible text for evidence of both the personality features and the experiences which are felt to be alien and which can be described as symptoms.

For the first clue we must return to the Prologue. Satan has just caused all of Job's children as well as his material possessions to be destroyed, and God points out to Satan that Job still retains his integrity. Satan replies:

> "Skin for skin! There is nothing the man will grudge to save himself. But stretch out your hand and touch his bone and flesh, and see if he will not curse you to your face."   (2: 4–5)

The metaphor "skin for skin" is relevant to a consideration of psychosomatic disorders which are concerned with body functions and body boundaries. The skin is the borderland between the individual and the outside world, where all his interactions are represented. Job's condition of running sores, which some medical commentators have equated with eczema,[16] is the *body's* first recognition (before *mental* recognition) that something is amiss. Although, as the Bible states, "Throughout all this, Job did not utter one sinful word" (2: 10), his body is already speaking for him; the damaged and broken skin represents the onset of Job's breakdown.

It is at this point that the three comforters enter the scene:

> When Job's three friends, Eliphaz of Teman, Bildad of Shuah, and Zophar of Naamah, heard of all these calamities which had overtaken him, they left their homes and arranged to come and condole with him and comfort him. But when they first saw him from a distance, they did not recognize him; and they wept aloud, rent their cloaks and tossed dust into the air over their heads. For seven

---

[16] For a discussion of other studies relating Job's illness to eczema and allied dermatological conditions, see Chapter 1, pp. 8–9.

days and seven nights they sat beside him on the ground, and none of them said
a word to him; for they saw that his suffering was very great.   (2: 11–13)

They find Job physically and mentally a changed man ("they did not
recognize him"). They share his dejection, first by weeping and tearing
their clothes, next by sitting beside him on the ground, and finally by
keeping a silence with him. They act out the grief that Job must be experiencing. Job's friends are subsequently given very little credit for his
recovery, but this act of identification is the first indication of group
support and interaction which will finally provide Job with the resources
with which he will construct his cure.

Outward posture is important as a reflection of the inner state of mind.
At the first calamity, Job "fell *prostrate* on the ground" (1: 21). This is an
act of acceptance and piety, bordering on the ritualistic. When the integrity
of his skin was broken into, he "*sat* among the ashes" (2: 8). This is a
position from which one may eventually "take stock" of a situation.[17]
This was where his friends find him. Job's state of mind and body is
completely different from that which was described as "blameless [perfect]
and *upright*" (1: 1). Job will remain seated until finally he reaches the stage
when God exhorts him to "*stand up* like a man".

In the opening words of chapter 3, Job finds expression for his anger.
His wish is to obliterate his own life, and his anger quickly turns to the
world outside him for having allowed him to be born. He is ready to
eclipse nature in order to erase the memory of his own existence:

> Perish the day when I was born
> and the night which said, 'A man is conceived'!
> May that day turn to darkness; may God above not look for it,
> nor light of dawn shine on it.
> May blackness sully it, and murk and gloom,
> cloud smother that day, swift darkness eclipse its sun.
> Blind darkness swallow up that night;   (3: 3–6)

It is a poetic device in drama and mythology to equate the creativity of
nature with human birth, and the mood of depression with darkness and

---

[17] In *The Magic Mountain*, Thomas Mann makes continued use of the semi-seated,
semi-reclining position from which the hero, Hans Castorp, sick in mind and body,
"takes stock" of his situation. From this position it eventually becomes possible
for him to go through certain emotional experiences which lead to what could be
considered his cure.

death. Job's regret that he came into existence makes him wish to deny any joy that his parents might have felt in his birth. He asks:

> Why was I ever laid on my mother's knees
> or put to suck at her breasts?   (3: 12)

The Authorized Version and the Soncino translation read as follows:

> Why did the knees prevent me?
> or why the breast that I should suck?

The Soncino Version supplies a footnote to the effect that the knees are those of the father who receive the child as a gesture of the acceptance of paternity.[18] The New English Version is an interesting variant in that it gratuitously attributes the knees to the mother. In either case, however, the knees stand as the symbol of acceptance, and, by the same token, Job repudiates whichever parent it was who had provided his legitimization.

In his declamations, Job is reversing ordinary values. He began with the theme of light as against dark; and he preferred the dark:

> May no star shine out in its twilight;
> may it wait for a dawn that never comes,
>   (3: 9)

The next theme is of life in the outside as against life in the womb; and he would have preferred life to have continued in the womb:

> . . . it did not shut the doors of the womb that bore me
> and keep trouble away from my sight.   (3: 10)

A further progression in this reversal of ordinary values is in the theme of life itself as against death during birth; and he would have preferred to be still-born:

> Why was I not still-born,
> why did I not die when I came out of the womb?
> . . .
> Why was I not hidden like an untimely birth,
> like an infant that has not lived to see the light?
>   (3: 11, 16)

---

[18] Soncino Books of the Bible: *Job*, p. 11.

His sufferings are so great that nothing in life could be made worthwhile. This is the depth of depression; it is the worthlessness of all that one is, of all that one still has, and of all that has gone before. It is even the worthlessness of that which one has lost.

Job goes on to ask the question,

> Why should the sufferer be born to see the light?
> Why is life given to men who find it so bitter?
> They wait for death but it does not come,
>
> (3: 20–21)

Here Job goes from his own particular case to a generalization—a generalization which has its modern counterpart in the discussions regarding the preservation of life in those who are born mentally or physically handicapped. Some of these might die but for the medical attention which is lavished on them. Even though they sometimes live to be a burden to themselves and to their families, the doctor feels that he has no alternative but to offer the knowledge and care that is within his possession.

There is a similar ethical consideration within the context of treating those suffering from depression and who are in danger of bringing their own life to an end. A psychiatrist is authorized to intervene, forcibly if necessary, in order to prevent suicide. And yet there is another dimension of treatment in which the therapist always aims at reflecting problems back to the patient together with an interpretation of them. In this dimension, it is for the patient to take subsequent responsibility for his actions, whatever these might be. Notwithstanding this, the duty to save life predominates, and is justified by the fact that many who have attempted suicide are able to survive and to gain and give some satisfaction in the remainder of their life. There are others, no doubt, who renew their depression and have to undergo their sufferings one or many times more. The doctor who saves life can give no guarantee that the life will be worthwhile. In like manner, there is the assumption (which some people challenge) that an infant's life must be preserved no matter what his life might become.[19] At the depths of his depression, Job had no reason to

---

[19] At some stage in the treatment of depression, or in the counselling of the parents of a handicapped child, the question might be asked: "What parts of your experience are there in which you have found some satisfaction?", or, more specifically, "What is there that has been good?"

think that his life could become any better. One might ask what it was that gave the comforters the justification for remaining with him through-out his silence and for engaging him in argument once the silence was broken.

Job turns from anger towards his parents to anger towards God. He blames God for his symptoms:

> The arrows of the Almighty find their mark in me,
> and their poison soaks into my spirit;
> God's onslaughts wear me away.   (6: 4)

Within the context of the Biblical story, Job is right. It was God who gave Satan the permission to cause the calamities and then the sore boils. If we were to limit our interpretations of Job's condition to his own com-munications, we could conclude that his accusation against the Almighty was the beginning of his ideas of being persecuted—the symptoms of paranoia. But a diagnosis of paranoia depends upon the delusional nature of the idea of persecution. Within the allegorical framework of the Pro-logue, God is in the wrong and Job is both innocent and justifiably aggrieved, since God had stated to Satan, "You incited me to ruin him without a cause" (2: 3).

At another level, what Job is expressing is consistent with traditional descriptions of depression. Aubrey Lewis finds a cause of depression in recent misfortunes in the patient's life:

> Any calamity to which human beings are liable may provoke an affective break-down . . . morbid depression following bereavement, financial setbacks or degradation.[20]

The loss of Job's children, the loss of his possessions, and the subsequent loss of his stature within his community, are followed by symptoms similar to those Lewis describes as occurring in depression:

> Delusions occur in proportion to the depth of affect; . . . The delusions are the product of the depression, which is primary . . . anxiety is prominent. Wicked-ness . . . loss of property . . . mortal or corrupting disease—these are the common substance of delusions and are often commingled. . . . The delusions may be grandiose in that the patient affirms himself the chief of sinners,[21] . . . or they may be of a minimising sort—nobody cares about him, he is of no account, let

---

[20] Aubrey Lewis, *op. cit.*, p. 1835.
[21] In Job's case, the "perfect" victim.

him go into a corner to hide, people despise him. This last belief is often understandably associated with ideas of reference or persecution—people make con-
temptuous gestures or remarks as he passes, they set detectives to watch him,
they tell each other how bad he is. . . . Many depressed patients, professing
humility, are importunate in their demands on those around them.[22]

At this point Job's complaints turn from descriptions of mental anguish
to the physical symptoms which he attributes to the onslaughts of God.
He has digestive disturbances:

> Food that should nourish me sticks in my throat,
> and my bowels rumble with an echoing sound.
>
> (6: 7)

The Soncino and Authorized Versions use the word "soul":

> The things that my soul refused to touch are as
> my sorrowful meat.

Whereas the New English translation of this verse puts a purely physical
connotation, the Authorized and Soncino Versions contrast soul and
flesh (meat). In Hebrew, the word for soul is often used for appetite. In
this context, it means that Job's whole being revolts against the food that
he needs for his physical nourishment.

Job refers to his sleepless night. He has insomnia:

> When the evening grows long and I lie down,
> I do nothing but toss till morning twilight.
>
> (7: 4)

the running sores are now scabbed over:

> My body is infested with worms,
> and scabs cover my skin.   (7: 5)

The nights are long with sleeplessness and the days are short, as is usual
with the depressed individual who revives in the afternoon but cannot face
the night:

> When I lie down, I think,
> "When will it be day that I may rise?"
>
> . . .
>
> My days are swifter than a shuttle
> and come to an end as the thread runs out.
>
> (7: 4, 6)

---

[22] Aubrey Lewis, *op. cit.*, p. 1885.

Job believes that he will never again return to his former good fortune:

> So months of futility are my portion,
> troubled nights are my lot.   (7: 3)

In periods of despair, it is impossible to believe that anything good will ever happen again. Life is all on one low level. There is no confidence in a better future—or in any future. Moreover, Job does not believe in an after-life which would compensate for his present troubles:

> As clouds break up and disperse,
> so he that goes down to Sheol never comes back;
>
> (7: 9)

Job's report of his physical condition tallies with Aubrey Lewis's description of the physical effects of depression:

> Sleep is bad—hard to come by, light and unrefreshing. The appetite is bad too; food may be constantly refused for this reason. Commonly also the patient eats too little because of feelings of fullness and other discomfort in the abdomen, or because of delusions about his bowels or his food. Mild constipation is common, but is often given much exaggerated importance by the patient. The weight diminishes, chiefly, but not by any means wholly, because of insufficient intake of food. Daily fluctuation in the general condition, with improvement towards evening is common. The skin may be dry and sallow, and in some severe cases pigmented, as it is in pellagra.[23]

A new element in the symptoms appears at this point. We have already noted that Job had accused God of persecuting him. The feeling of persecution from the outside now takes a specific form. The paranoid process has identified the persecutors as living individuals who are the agents of God. Addressing God, Job asks why "thou settest a watch over me" (7: 12), and this implies that the three comforters, who have indeed given him very little comfort, were planted there by God to watch over Job.

Job accuses God of sending him terrifying dreams and frightening visions, so that he can find no comfort even in his sleep:

> When I think that my bed will comfort me,
> that sleep will relieve my complaining,
> thou dost terrify me with dreams
> and affright me with visions.   (7: 13–14)

---

[23] *Ibid*, p. 1886.

He looks to death as an escape from this torment:

> I would prefer death to all my sufferings.
> I am in despair, I would not go on living;
>   (7: 15–16)

Death is an escape and a refuge:

> But now I shall lie down in the grave;
> seek me, and I shall not be.   (7: 21)

Job's God had previously been a just God because Job had enjoyed good fortune in return for his righteousness. Now that Job's fortunes have changed, God's attributes have also changed. Job now sees him as being too strong:

> It is God who moves mountains, giving them no rest,
> turning them over in his wrath;   (9: 5)

He is too busy:

> he moves on his way undiscerned by me;
> if he hurries on, who can bring him back?
>   (9: 11–12)

He is unjust:

> Though I am right, I get no answer,
> though I plead with my accuser for mercy.
>   (9: 15)

He is persecuting:

> he leaves me no respite to recover my breath
> but fills me with bitter thoughts.   (9: 18)

He is capricious:

> But it is all one; therefore I say,
> 'He destroys blameless and wicked alike.'
>   (9: 22)

He is mocking:

> When a sudden flood brings death,
> he mocks the plight of the innocent.
> (9: 23)

The attributes can be considered as part of human thoughts about the nature of God, but at an individual level it could be considered as representing a stage in which Job's breakdown gives him the freedom to venture dangerous thoughts which in his normal state would have remained concealed. In the development of the idea of God, Job will change his views once again. In the meantime, it is worth noting that the ambivalence which Job has been shown to feel in his personal relationship with, for example, his children has now been extended to include hostility towards God.

The persecutory nature of the list of attributes which Job attaches to God are relevant to traditional descriptions of the symptomatology of paranoia. In Henderson and Gillespie's *Textbook*, symptoms of paranoia are described as follows:

> These patients brood over grievances, and then project and rationalize their aggression, hatred or longing. Ideas of reference insidiously become delusions of persecution. Plots, they believe, are hatched against them: their thoughts, their persons and their property are interfered with.[24]

Job returns to his symptoms. He says, "I tremble in every nerve" (9: 28). He has good reason to tremble. If God has all the attributes that Job ascribes to him, it would be ineffectual for Job to deny the guilt which was imputed to him by the comforters or even by his own unbidden thoughts. All that remains for him is to attempt to wash it away:

> Though I wash myself with soap
> or cleanse my hands with lye,
> thou wilt thrust me into the mud
> and my clothes will make me loathsome.
> (9: 30–31)

We have already implied that the diagnosis of a single clinical syndrome is an artificial construct onto the manifold human experiences of mental

[24] *Henderson & Gillespie's Textbook of Psychiatry*, rev. by Ivor Batchelor, 10th ed (London: Oxford University Press, 1969), p. 295.

disorder, and here we have obsessional features added to the depression and the paranoia.

With depression goes anger against nature. With obsessional states, the aim is to bring it under control. The notion is that a ritual can change the order of nature, can undo what has been done, or prevent what is due to occur. Washing can wash away internal guilt and ritual prayers can command God.

But there is a contradiction. Job acknowledges his impotence in his efforts to control the outcome, yet he still claims an understanding equal with God of the forces that are unfairly arrayed against him:

> Yet this was the secret purpose of thy heart,
> and I know that this was thy intent:
> that, if I sinned, thou wouldst be watching me
> and wouldst not acquit me of my guilt.
> . . .
> thou dost renew thy onslaught upon me,
> and with mounting anger against me
> bringest fresh forces to the attack.
>
> (10: 13–17)

The ideas of persecution begin to dominate him, and he addresses God directly, asserting that God created him merely in order to persecute him. Jung makes the point that it was with God's foreknowledge that Job's sufferings were initiated.[25] If God had consulted his omniscience, he would have known what the results would be. Job himself makes the same point, namely that his sufferings were deliberately inflicted. How could it be otherwise, as God knew in advance what would happen? Goodness or badness would make no difference. Job's suffering was prejudged:

> If I indeed am wicked, the worse for me!
> If I am righteous, even so I may lift up my head;
> if I am proud as a lion, thou dost hunt me down
> and dost confront me again with marvellous power;
>
> (10: 15–16)

Job returns to his former lamentations by renouncing his birth and regretting his post-natal existence:

[25] Carl Jung, *Answer to Job*, trans. R. F. C. Hull (London: Hodder & Stoughton, 1964).

Why didst thou bring me out of the womb?
O that I had ended there and no eye had seen me,
that I had been carried from the womb to the grave
and were as though I had not been born.

(10: 18–19)

Job seeks to alleviate his distress, but there is no way in which he can find relief:

If I speak, my pain is not eased;
if I am silent, it does not leave me.

(16: 6)

He describes the way in which he feels that he is being attacked:

My enemies look daggers at me,
they bare their teeth to rend me,
they slash my cheeks with knives;
they are all in league against me.
God has left me at the mercy of malefactors
and cast me into the clutches of wicked men.

(16: 10–11)

These are the words of one who feels to be the object of conspiracy. It is the language of paranoia.

It could be argued that this description is no more than an exaggerated figure of speech, intended to describe persecutions which Job feels to be real. The diagnosis of paranoia is made when there is objective evidence that the persecution is not real. And yet even when someone genuinely suffers from discrimination, a diagnosis of paranoia might still be made on the basis of the manner and quality of his complaint. Within different cultures, there are variations in the amount of exaggeration which is acceptable when making a complaint. The use of metaphor has its conventions and boundaries. Sometimes the abnormal nature of the complaint is recognized by the way it enhances the importance of the one to whom the attacks are directed. Job considers himself specially selected by God:

He set me up as his target;
his arrows rained upon me from every side;
pitiless, he cut deep into my vitals,

(16: 12–13)

The greater Job's misfortunes, the greater becomes his image of himself.

Job begins to imagine somebody greater than God who could intercede between God and Job:

> If only there were one to arbitrate between man and God,
> (16: 21)

Once Job has a conception of someone greater than God, he has challenged the ultimate qualities of the deity: the omnipotence, the omniscience, and the perfection of ideals that go with God's knowledge and power. These qualities have to pass to the one who would be the arbitrator. God has become smaller, and Job has become larger as the disputing partner in the arbitration. This is exaltation which now emerges out of the depression.

The exalted mood soon gives way; depression returns:

> my eyes are dim with grief,
> my limbs wasted to a shadow.
> (17: 7)

Job has been contemplating suicide. He is taking his thoughts into the physical experience of the approach of death:

> My days die away like an echo;
> my heart-strings are snapped.
> (17: 11)

Job now makes friends with death and seeks comfort in it. In death he hopes to find a home:

> If I measure Sheol for my house,
> if I spread my couch in the darkness,
> if I call the grave my father
> and the worm my mother or my sister,
> where, then, will my hope be,
> and who will take account of my piety?
> (17: 13–15)

He is surrounding himself with the idea of death, even, tentatively, contemplating death as a return to a home which he had once enjoyed and had lost. He realizes, however, that, as with his material possessions, he cannot take his virtues with him into death:

> I cannot take them down to Sheol with me,
> nor can they descend with me into the earth.
> (17: 16)

Like Hamlet, his reluctance to commit suicide rests on the notion that the after-life may be as imperfect as the present one. He cannot even take with him his one remaining possession—his undiminished piety.

Job's preoccupation with death gives way to accusations against the people around him:

> How long will you exhaust me
> and pulverize me with words?
> Time and time again you have insulted me
> and shamelessly done me wrong.
>
> (19: 2–3)

He feels that his friends have ignored his real needs at the time when he most needed comfort. Their long speeches are an insult to his suffering:

> If I cry "Murder!" no one answers;
> if I appeal for help, I get no justice.
>
> (19: 7)

By their insensitiveness, they deny him the help for which he is appealing. No one comes to his aid to save his life, or his repute. From this he goes on to describe the way in which all his former associates have purposely excluded him from their love and from their company:

> My brothers hold aloof from me,
> my friends are utterly estranged from me;
> my kinsmen and intimates fall away,
> my retainers have forgotten me;
> my slave-girls treat me as a stranger,
> I have become an alien in their eyes.
> I summon my slave, but he does not answer,
> though I entreat him as a favour.
> My breath is noisome to my wife,
> and I stink in the nostrils of my own family.
> Mere children despise me
> and, when I rise, turn their backs on me;
> my intimate companions loathe me,
> and those whom I love have turned against me.
> My bones stick out through my skin,
> and I gnaw my under-lip with my teeth.
>
> (19: 13–20)

Job feels abhorrent to his family and friends—and there is good cause for the feeling of revulsion which they show. With depression often comes loss ppetite, and lack of eating and drinking leads to bad-smelling breath. There is evidence that he is ill-nourished, in that he is so thin that his "bones stick out through [his] skin".

The physical and mental aspects of his symptoms are intermingled here. The Authorized Version offers a well-quoted figure of speech, "I have escaped with the skin of my teeth" (19: 20), whereas the New English Version renders it literally ("I gnaw my under-lip with my teeth"). The Soncino commentary on this verse concludes that Job's "entire body is ravaged with disease, even his teeth have fallen out and he is left with the bare gums."[26] Freudian and other dynamic schools of psychology attach significance to the use of imagery connected with eating and biting. Without going into some of the depths of analytical interpretation, it can be noted that people are described figuratively as being "eaten up with hate", and that the paranoid person can feel that he is being literally "eaten up by others".

The language of eating and being eaten continues when Job begs his comforters for mercy:

> Pity me, pity me, you that are my friends;
> for the hand of God has touched me.
> Why do you pursue me as God pursues me?
> Have you not had your teeth in me long enough?
> (19: 21–22)

It is difficult to tell whether Job is using a metaphor or whether he is describing, as if it were literally true, what he experiences. The difference is important in distinguishing between psychosis and neurosis. The psychotic person says, "My brain is eaten away", while the neurotic person says, "I feel *as if* my brain were eaten away". Either way, Job is now accusing his friends of persecuting him in the same manner as God had done.

Again Job passes from complaining of being the victim of persecution to giving vent to ideas of boastful self-importance:

> O that my words might be inscribed,
> O that my words might be engraved in an inscription,
> to be a witness in hard rock! (19: 23–24)

He feels that his suffering is so important that it is worthy of being inscribed for preservation in perpetuity (which is exactly what happened).

[26] Soncino Version, *op. cit.*, p. 98.

The self-importance of his former character endures through his illness and has survived the depression. In so far as he was a great man, his suffering is of great importance.

His feeling of being persecuted by God returns:

> He decides, and who can turn him from his purpose?
> He does what his own heart desires.
> What he determines, that he carries out;
> his mind is full of plans like these.
> Therefore I am fearful of meeting him;
> it is God who makes me faint-hearted
> and the Almighty who fills me with fear,
>
> (23: 13–16)

Here the imagery is confused, but Job's state of mind somewhat resembles that of a child who looks upon the distinguishing characteristic of the adult as being able to do exactly what he wants. Job is the child and God represents the adult. There is also a political analogy. In a totalitarian state, those who are in power can do exactly what they wish and govern their actions by the way the governed fulfil expectations which had never been made manifest. Job claims that God is not consistent, and therefore he cannot figure out what he should do in order to satisfy him. This is a Kafkaesque theme where one inevitably is judged to be wrong without knowing what it is that one has done. There is always a "catch" which serves the purpose of putting the weaker person in the wrong. The catch inherent in the child–adult relationship is that the adult is felt by the child to be omnipotent and omniscient, without imparting the power and knowledge which he possesses. Aims and purposes, rights and wrongs, are never clearly defined. The child may feel that he will gain mastery of this knowledge and power when he is adult, but not even maturity gives the right to the gifts which have been held out to the child and then denied.

For a brief spell Job turns his thoughts to the good old days, like a child returning to its mother after a separation. This is an acknowledgement for the first time that the previous life was not all bad.

> If I could only go back to the old days,
> to the time when God was watching over me,
> when his lamp shone above my head,
> and by its light I walked through the darkness!
>
> (29: 2–3)

but immediately the symptoms return—and for the last time:

> Terror upon terror overwhelms me,
> it sweeps away my resolution like the wind,
> and my hope of victory vanishes like a cloud.
> So now my soul is in turmoil within me,
> and misery has me daily in its grip.
> By night pain pierces my very bones,
> and there is ceaseless throbbing in my veins;
> my garments are all bespattered with my phlegm,
> which chokes me like the collar of a shirt.
> God himself has flung me down in the mud,
> no better than dust or ashes.   (30: 15-19)

As frequently occurs in the penultimate crisis of therapy, the first symptoms reappear almost as if there were a deliberate attempt to preserve the memory of an illness which has passed its zenith:

> My bowels are in ferment and know no peace;
> days of misery stretch out before me.
> I go about dejected and friendless;
> . . .
> My blackened skin peels off,   (30: 27-30)

The symptoms had subsided, or, in so far as they persisted, they had become of less importance to Job, until the climax where Job is about to achieve a new stage of development.

CHAPTER 4

The Case for Treatment

WE believe that we have made a case in the first section for dealing with Job's experiences as an illness. It is now our purpose to trace the events and processes to which the term "therapy" could be applied. This chapter, and the two subsequent ones, will be concerned with the course of Job's illness and its treatment. The division into chapters is artificial. The themes are intricately linked.

In order to consider Job's illness in terms of therapy, we must bring in a dimension other than the one in which the story is told. The original framework is the cultural and religious one, and, ostensibly, it concerns a man who was tested by God in a wager with Satan, who survived the test (at least in the first place), and who later rebelled. He had comforters whose standing within the story was a natural part of the cultural background in which the story was told. He was restored to his health and fortune through the intervention of God.

We shall alter this framework by giving a naturalistic explanation of Job's experiences, and, for this purpose, we shall treat the religious framework as only part—although a very important part—of the influences which impinge upon the mind of an individual. We shall therefore need to examine the events portrayed in the story under a conceptual system different from that in which the original events are portrayed.

There are a number of ways of looking upon what happens to Job.

Human beings have studied themselves in terms of philosophy and religion. The story of Job has received ample consideration from these points of view, and, although there is always something new to be discovered in any chosen dimension, these are outside the purview of this book.

There are also portrayals of human events in the framework of drama, where a whole action sequence is reduced to a few basic themes, and where one central character may have his life presented on the stage by the dramatist in relation to its impact on the lives of other characters. In Greek drama there is an inevitability of a tragic outcome, given the basic premises of the story. Conversely, a present-day dramatist might wish to demonstrate the fact that the outcome, whatever it may be, comes by chance. Thus, in one case the aim is to show purpose and meaning in a pre-determined sequence; in the other it is the purposelessness and meaning-lessness of life that is portrayed. Drama is, in this respect, an attempt to give a general view of life, and dramatic techniques are the means by which people and events are handled in order to bring about a conclusion which is desired and/or feared. Drama, in common with other art forms, is a human activity based upon intuition, in which a fragment of human conduct and experience is presented in a way in which the action can be shared vicariously by others. The selection which is made for presentation is in itself an interpretation of the importance of the action.

Drama thus becomes one of the alternatives within a psychological framework. It could be broadened to include other art forms, such as poetry, music, and the plastic arts. We have already referred to Blake's drawings of Job, MacLeishe's *J.B.*, and we could mention, in passing, Vaughan Williams's *Job: A Masque for Music*.

The psychodynamic interpretation is a statement within psychology in which there is an aim to effect change. It embraces many schools of study. The life history of an individual is seen generally as the outcome of the interaction of the individual's conscious and unconscious inner forces, and the relationship with his environment. Within this framework, the following factors may be differentially stressed: developmental progress of the individual from birth onwards; beneficial and harmful experiences occurring at each stage of life; constitutional inheritance; critical events in the life cycle; interpersonal relationships in the family or larger group-ings; the general level of support available, both informally and through organized services. This dimension also takes into account the prevailing values within the culture, whether materialistic, religious, political, aesthetic, etc.

The psychodynamic dimension, with its therapeutic implications, allows us to take all the recorded circumstances as factors in Job's illness and his recovery, whether they were intended for that purpose or not. It also gives us freedom to consider the therapeutic situation and the therapeutic process in terms of Job's inner mental processes and in terms of his interactions with the group that forms around him.

What we have as evidence of the course of Job's illness is a number of speeches set in a manner more appertaining to a dramatic than a psychotherapeutic framework. Our own task requires the translation of these communications into the idiom of dynamic psychology, laying aside the religious, philosophical, historical, and physical interpretations. The speeches are our evidence of Job's experiences: the losses which he suffered, his symptoms, and the means by which he recovered his health, wealth, and family, and achieved further personal growth.

The description of the course of the illness cannot be separated from the consideration of the nature of the cure. This is an essential part of our approach. When a patient gives an account of an illness, he changes the course of that illness. When anyone puts his feelings into words, with other people responding, there is a reshaping of the experience that is being described. Each communication is a way of construing an experience inside the person. The construction becomes the property of those who share in the communication and becomes altered in the process. People commit themselves to views, and, having committed themselves, they and their views are open to challenge. The communication of the view is a form of action, and the very describing of feelings or of symptoms becomes a form of behaviour in which change is possible.

We are assuming that all Job's transactions with the comforters, Elihu, and God, have an effect, as well as an affect, both of which have to be interpreted. It is only possible by hindsight to say that the outcome of the story of Job is influenced by the series of transactions which take place. Our interpretations are made in the full knowledge of the positive nature of the outcome. However, Job himself had no reason to assume this. Indeed, he believed the opposite to be true—that his misfortunes, sufferings, and persecutions would continue indefinitely in the future.

It will be our thesis that it was his very protest against the deterministic explanation of his suffering that made Job alter the outcome of his illness.

Had he remained within the religious convention, he would have had to agree that his suffering was the punishment for past sins. One can find times during the course of the Book when he entertains that possibility. Yet his main contention was a challenge to this view. Being unable to admit that he was less than perfect, he was compelled—or one might say doomed—to make the discovery of a view of human suffering that lay outside the prevailing philosophy and religious teaching. His stimulus to search for new explanations was bound up with his undying contention that he had not sinned. If he had accepted his guilt, he would have had to submit to his fate. The Prologue could well have been invented at this point by Job himself:[1] God did not impose Job's suffering within a deterministic system of reward and punishment. It was a wager between Satan and God, in which the stake was Job's fate.

Job had barely survived, but he was ready to demand that God should renew the wager—this time with Job himself—the stake being God's reputation for justice. In this, as we shall show later, Job was challenging outmoded religious conceptions and, at the same time, he was taking his suffering out of the religious framework. He was preparing the way for the construction of his cure.

The above formulation allows us to return to our own consideration of a naturalistic explanation of Job's illness: its causation, its symptoms, and its cure. The particular point which we must emphasize here is that the calamities were a *loss* to Job, and the predominant initial feature of his illness was depressive. The experience of loss and consequent depression brought the comforters to Job's side. Only in the presence of these comforters could Job have developed the ideas which carried him through a number of processes after his initial withdrawal; to self-recrimination; to anger; and then to a paranoid state in which the persecution was projected onto outside sources. If, during all this, Job preserved some of the obsessional features of his personality, these provided him with the strength to keep himself intact. In his rebellion he was able to find the material for reconstructing the personality which he had preserved.

In modern clinical psychiatry the treatment is given shape according to the way in which the illness is perceived. In this case the illness is envisaged as having depressive, obsessional, and paranoid features. This forms the

[1] God says to Satan: "You incited me to ruin him *without a cause*" (2: 3), and later Job complains that God "rains blows on me *without cause*" (9: 17).

prototype for the structure which we are creating out of the Bible narrative. Next we draw upon the responses and interactions of Job with the three original comforters and with Elihu. This is the practical aspect (the therapeutic situation). Finally, what is presented in the Biblical text as the appearance of God is being considered for our purposes as taking place within the mind of Job, and it is in the mind of Job that we can locate the process of cure.

We have referred to the links between the premorbid personality and the morbid condition (the illness). It would be equally true to say that there are features in the premorbid personality which serve the therapeutic process. Some of these features are best described in non-medical language, as drawn directly from the Bible text, and it is only the clinical inferences about the origin of these features in someone's life history, and purposes they serve, which call for technical terms.

We have described Job as having an "obsessional personality", in that he made an attempt to influence external events by his religious observances and his "perfect" behaviour. Freud traced obsessional symptoms to a reversal of the aim of an instinct from active to passive form, and noted that obstinacy and stubbornness were prominent character traits.[2] When Elihu spoke of pride and stubbornness, he was referring to the same qualities which gave Job his claim to perfection. Fenichel, dealing with obsessional personality in a psychoanalytical framework, offers a description of stubbornness which could well have fitted Elihu's allusions to Job:

> Originally, stubbornness meant only resistance, to pit one's will against somebody else; later, it meant pitting one's own will against superior inimical forces; still later (because the inimical forces are superior), getting one's way indirectly, not through force but through guile, in a mode wherein the weak one may be unexpectedly strong. Stubbornness is a passive type of aggressiveness, developed where activity is impossible. . . . What is usually called stubbornness in the behaviour of adult persons is an attempt to use other persons as instruments in the struggle with the super-ego. . . .
>
> The moral superiority may be experienced either through the feeling of being unfairly treated itself or through making the "unfair" adult sorry afterward, which should enforce affection from him.
>
> In other words, stubbornness, initially the combative method of the weak,

---

[2] Dr. Humberto Nagera *et al.*, *Basic Psychoanalytic Concepts on the Libido Theory* (London: Ruskin House, 1969), p. 29.

later becomes the habitual combative method in the struggle for the mainten-
ance or the restoration of self-esteem. . . .[3]

Here the obsessional personality is seen as a construction which is de-
signed to reconcile rebellion and obedience. When Job calls God to
account for his suffering on the basis that he had always led a perfect and
blameless life, he is rebelling within an accepted mode of obedience. Job
could argue God out of court on the basis of having led his life according
to the rules laid down in Deuteronomy and Leviticus.

> Since most patriarchal religions also veer between submission to a paternal
> figure and rebellion (both submission and rebellion being sexualized), and every
> god, like a compulsive superego, promises protection on condition of submis-
> sion, there are many similarities in the manifest picture of compulsive ceremon-
> ials and religious rituals, due to the similarity of the underlying conflicts. Freud,
> therefore, has called a compulsion neurosis a private religion.[4]

Although the obsessional traits are seen to comply with accepted cultural demands, these traits appear to give to their possessor extra powers
which border on an omnipotence equal to that of God.

Job had enjoyed many years of prosperity during which he maintained
his religious observances. His belief in their efficacy was continually reinforced so long as his fortunes and his stature within his community were
maintained. The loss of his possessions suddenly deprived him of the
evidence which confirmed him in his religious practices. His concept of
himself and his idea of his own identity as the greatest man in the East
were destroyed by external events. Job then became the victim of internal
conflicting forces.

Many of the theoretical ideas which we are selecting for our therapeutic framework here and previously are derived from classical psychoanalytical sources. Alternative formulations can be found in some of the
newer psychological and sociological writings. Taking the description of
Job as "blameless and upright" and as the "greatest man in the East", we
can draw inferences from Laing's concept of a "pivotal self-definition":

> Let us suppose that something happens that is incompatible with the nuclear
> pivotal definition ["perfect and upright"] . . . that . . . is determining the in-

---

[3] Otto Fenichel, *The Psychoanalytic Theory of Neurosis* (New York: W. W.
Norton & Co., 1945), pp. 279–280.

[4] *Ibid.*, pp. 301–302.

dividual's whole system of meanings. It is as though a linch-pin has been removed that had been holding the person's whole world together. Something has happened that challenges the whole meaning that the individual has been giving to "reality". It "takes the ground from under" his feet. At least temporarily, that mode of participation in the world that we denote by such terms as "contact with" and "sense of reality" is stripped of validity. What is left is the primary level of phantasy. That person will be plunged into a most desperate crisis, where either he must restructure his whole "real" view of others and the world and hence, basically, redefine his "real" self; or he may try to annul the chasm between his definition of himself and the way others define him, by taking his stand on a self-definition whose basis is the primary experience of what we are calling phantasy.[5]

The loss of this self-identification, which was one more loss added to the others, was the occasion for the disturbance of Job's physical health and mental balance. The attack on Job's integrity is symbolized by physical symptoms and by grief.

Grief takes a form in which the depressive process has inner and outer targets and the degree to which the anger accompanying grief is turned against the outside in some cases of acute mourning is a measure of the inner anger which had already existed.

> . . . far from evincing towards those around them the attitude of humility and submission . . . they give a great deal of trouble, perpetually taking offence and behaving as if they had been treated with great injustice.[6]

In an unconscious way, the obsessionally neurotic individual imbues his rituals with the power to control fate, thus investing himself with omnipotent-like qualities. The depressed person has carried these unconscious phantasies of influence over the fate of others into his feelings in mourning the death of someone significant to him. He is ready to find a way in which some act of commission or omission on his part was responsible for that death. Job was continually offering sacrifices in order to preserve the lives of his children. Why, then, did they die? The distress during the mourning is a turning in of the anger which followed the failure of the obsessional techniques. It would take only one further step from this internalized anger to the state of paranoia in which the hostile forces within are envisaged as being met by similar forces from the outside world. The link between obsession, depression, and paranoia can be seen in

[5] R. D. Laing, The Self and Others (London: Tavistock Publications, 1961), p. 82.
[6] Sigmund Freud, "Mourning and melancholia", op. cit., p. 248.

phantasies concerning the ability to influence people and events by the power of thought; or, conversely, in the phantasies that other people possess similar powers over the self.

Vacillation between depressive and paranoid processes has been discussed by Melanie Klein:

> The stronger the neurosis of the child, the less he is able to effect that transition to the depressive position [from the persecutory], and its working through is impeded by a vacillation between persecutory and depressive anxiety. Throughout this early development, a regression to the paranoid-schizoid stage may take place, whereas a stronger ego and a greater capacity to bear suffering results in a greater insight into his psychic reality and enables him to work through the depressive position.[7]

The anger which Job turns against himself in his wish for self-annihilation turns to anger against God and the comforters. He in turn fears them as persecutory figures.

Alongside the vacillation Job maintains an enduring identity through reliance on his integrity—the superego which was expressed in his obsessional rituals and his acts of charity and generosity. This was the source of his reputation as the greatest man in the East.

The superego has often been described as if it were a separate entity acting within the individual. It embodies all the restrictions on conduct which are part of public and private religions and, even when an individual's actions are in opposition to the implied standards, some general harmony is maintained in which the superego forms an integral part of the concept of self-identity. The superego, however, may be experienced separately as a persecuting entity, imposing intolerable demands. This persecuting force may be transferred to outside figures.

When the whole basis of Job's conduct is called into question in relation to the ideal model within him, he perceives himself as being brought into opposition with an external persecuting superego which is his own projection as well as having a living embodiment in the persons of the comforters. As a projection, this is the root of paranoia.

> . . . these patients consider the outward establishment of their integrity and innocence as the most important thing in the world. Since this establishment is

---

[7] Melanie Klein, *Our Adult World and its Roots in Infancy* (London: William Heinemann, 1963), p. 28.

carried out through conflicts with courts and authorities, it is reasonable to assume that in this type of delusion, as in delusions of reference, there is a projection of the superego, particularly in its critical and punitive aspects. The salient feature in such cases is the hostile attitude towards the authority representing the superego. This hostility is based on an assumed self-security and overestimation of the patient's own person arising from the narcissistic regression.[8]

Paranoia is also concerned with the way in which individuals are excluded or exclude themselves from communities, organizations, and from the family. It is true that the paranoid person is unduly suspicious, and has identifiable delusions of persecution, but it is also important to realize that most of the delusions have some foundation. Exclusion is based on reality. Within the Biblical story, it is in fact a conspiratorial action between God and Satan against Job which brings upon Job's sufferings. It is also true that Job felt that the comforters did little to comfort him and much to undermine his position. Moreover, Job reported actions from those around which made him feel socially isolated:

> my kinsmen and intimates fall away,
> my slave-girls treat me as a stranger,
> I have become an alien in their eyes.
> (19: 14–15)

In the sense that the paranoid person is himself the source of the exclusion, we have the quarrelsome and litigious propensities:

> From the vantage of others the individual in the paranoid relationship shows:
> 1. A disregard for the values and norms of the primary group, revealed by giving priority to verbally definable values over those which are implicit, a lack of loyalty in return for confidences, and victimizing and intimidating persons in positions of weakness.
> 2. A disregard for the implicit structure of groups, revealed by presuming to privileges not accorded him, and the threat or actual resort to formal means for achieving his goals.[9]

Such individuals can often take cases up to the highest courts. This reliance on legalistic means is illustrated by Job's insistence upon taking God to court to prove himself in the right.

---

[8] Otto Fenichel, *op. cit.*, p. 433.
[9] E. M. Lemert, "Dynamics of exclusion" in T. J. Scheff (ed.), *Mental Illness and Social Processes* (New York: Harper & Row, 1967), p. 277.

Job really never succeeds in pinning down his accusers. But in this his position is comparable with that of the paranoid patient who in present-day practice is induced to accept psychiatric treatment. Such a patient feels that he is persecuted and maintains that the persecution is real. Those around him tell him that he is deluded, and the fault is within him—the fault in this case being illness. If the psychiatrist agrees with this conclusion, then, by denying the reality of the persecution, he is colluding with the persecutors. But however much the patient protests that he is not mentally ill, his very protest and physical struggles against those who restrain him are taken as further evidence of his insanity. He has to admit that his persecution is delusional in order eventually to be given a certificate of his sanity. The paranoid person is able to extricate himself from this position by finding some contact with the residual healthy part of his personality. Whenever there is sufficient good will in the therapeutic team which confronts the patient, some common ground can finally be found. The patient is given respect for the totality of his personality and this helps the patient on his part to find new interpretations for his experience.

In the new schools which give themselves the name of anti-psychiatry, emphasis is placed on the invidious position of the patient who is called paranoid when, in reality, he is persecuted not least by his therapist. In these writings[10] the nature of the mental illness is denied and the disjunction between the patient and others is presented as disease in the surrounding culture.

The therapeutic framework which we are assuming in the case of Job could contain all these diverse elements. A man who is unjustly treated by God, and who is distressed, is admonished by his comforters for the sin which might have justified the infliction of his suffering. Job asserts his sinlessness. In being offered the traditional dogmas by way of "comfort", he is in a position similar to that of the mentally disordered person who claims that he is sane but who is pressed to accept the formulations of the traditional psychiatry of his age.

We have indicated that the division between sanity and insanity is blurred, and that there is no need to take sides, attributing absolute sanity to the patient and insanity to the therapist (as representative of

[10] See, for example, Robert Boyers and Robert Orrill (Eds.), *Laing and Anti-Psychiatry* (London: Penguin Education, 1972).

society), or vice versa. The new anti-psychiatry, which makes the patient into the blameless victim of his social environment, is as prejudicial to his cure as the traditional psychiatry which assumes that all the pathology resides within him.

We shall try to trace the course of Job's illness, and its cure, to communications which are ambiguous and which allow for development of new meanings and new understanding of experiences and events. This process depends upon the therapeutic potential which remained in Job's personality. It finally found expression in God's words "out of the whirlwind". We are putting forward the idea that these words, like the Prologue, were in the mind of Job.

CHAPTER 5

The Therapeutic Situation

THE three men who came to be with Job in his suffering did so with the express purpose of comforting him. But they gave Job little comfort. Indeed, they did their utmost to aggravate his suffering by putting forward the view, again and again, that his misfortunes were proof that he had sinned. The hostility which they showed towards Job, almost from the outset, is part of the ambivalence of a long-standing relationship, the other component being the friendship which it was their intent to express.

When they arrive on the scene they find Job so changed as to be unrecognizable. Their first actions showed identification with Job in his grief: "they wept aloud, rent their cloaks and tossed dust into the air over their heads." They express their sympathy by acting out, in ritual, the inner feelings which they might have attributed to Job. At this stage the comforters impose neither their consolations nor their strictures upon Job. They keep silent with him for seven days and nights.

Many changes in mood must have taken place during the silence. Job was the first to reveal the thoughts and feelings which in conventional communications remain undisclosed.

The value of the comfort which Job's three friends gave to him was consistently underestimated by Job and, indeed, by most Bible commentators. But there can be no doubt that the presence of the comforters created a situation for Job pregnant with therapeutic and pathogenic possibilities. Together they form a group. Their common religious and ideological heritage is the basis for cohesion. Their separate strivings for individuality and their mutual hostility provide the disruptive element. These are the features which a group therapist utilizes in treatment.

The treatment began with their silence, which can be considered as a sympathetic identification with Job's situation. In descriptions of psychotherapy, it is often taken for granted that the therapeutic medium is verbal communication. But the silences are as important as the spoken messages, and it is the sympathetic and accepting silence of the therapist which frequently aids the patient in constructing his cure:

> The psychotherapeutic situation utilizes both the *horror vacui* and its specific "medication," a human relationship, as the therapist partially fills in the void by his support and encouragement while at the same time (and unconsciously) forcing the patient to move forward into anxiety.[1]

The silence of the comforters, matching the silence of Job, released the anger which had been concealed in Job's depression. Up to the breaking of the silence, Job "did not utter one sinful word." Neither did the comforters utter a word of reproach to Job.[2]

After the silence come the communications. The cycles of speeches form transactions which we shall look at collectively, as well as separately, in the continuation of Job's treatment.

We have suggested that Job and the three comforters form a therapeutic group. The comparison with a present-day psychotherapeutic group cannot be pushed too far. Such a group is formed artificially for the specific purpose of therapy. Moreover, a modern therapeutic group would consist of a number of participants, who are patients, and one leader who is considered, for the purposes of the group, as healthy. From that viewpoint, the group which forms around Job is an inverse group, with Job notionally as the only sick one and the comforters as the healthy ones.

There is evidence of an outer group who, although silent, would have been by no means inert. Elihu later implied that he had been a sensitive witness to all that had happened, and, up to his intervention, he must have been merely one of a number of participant observers.

[1] Harley C. Shands, "The war with words: creativity and success", in J. Masserman (Ed.), *Communication and Community* (New York: Grune & Stratton, 1965), p. 141.

[2] In this they differed from his wife, who had challenged the whole basis of Job's religious faith and way of life. Job's wife had reproached him for maintaining his perfection, granting him that the perfection existed and merely questioning its worth on a scale of everyday values. At a later stage, the comforters will come to question the reality of Job's original perfection.

Our own position is not entirely consistent, because, while looking upon Job as receiving treatment which leads to cure, we shall at times challenge the notion that he was the sick one and that the others were all healthy.

The group around Job came together spontaneously, and within the convention of the culture of the time. The basis of its formation was the accepted practice that those who undergo misfortune are entitled to the comfort of their friends, relatives, and neighbours.

The pattern of the speeches is stylized into three cycles, each comforter being allowed one speech per cycle, giving Job the opportunity to give his response to each. This structure allows Job to predominate, even though he is a single contender against many.

After the silence, Job has the first words; after God speaks, at the end of the Book, Job has the last word. In between, Job completes the three cycles after the comforters have been reduced to silence (a different silence) once again. It is only to the young man Elihu that Job has no answer; and Elihu will play a crucial part in the therapeutic process.

Having come to offer sympathy, the comforters soon lose patience with Job. This is because he refuses to accept their premises or to subscribe to the traditional views which they represent. He dares to rebel against his fate.

It is also true to say that in any case Job would be a difficult person to comfort. He was, after all, supposed to be the greatest man in the East; and his personality was such that he would be unable to accept comfort from his peers amongst whom he was always considered the first.

Job can no more relinquish his claim to integrity, righteousness, and superiority, than they can go beyond the accepted viewpoint of the time, namely that suffering is punishment for sins. They are the protagonists of the moral balance sheet: the idea that goodness is rewarded in kind and that sins are punished proportionately.

Such a view places Job in a position which has been called the "double bind".[3] If he accepts the comforters' thesis, then he has to admit that he has sinned and that the calamities which befell him were justified. To deny his guilt, on the other hand, is tantamount to rebelling against the traditional religious outlook of his time. Either way, to accept the stand-

[3] For a discussion of the double bind, see G. Bateson, D. D. Jackson, J. Haley, *et al.*, "Toward a theory of schizophrenia", *Behav. Sci.* **1** (1956), pp. 251–264.

What! shall we recieve Good
at the hand of God & shall we not also
recieve Evil

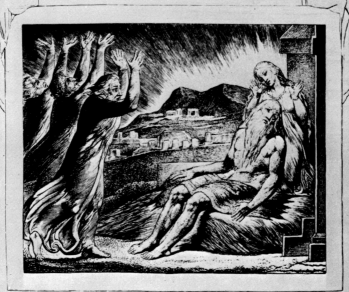

And when they lifted up their eyes afar off & knew him not
they lifted up their voice & wept. & they rent every Man his
mantle & sprinkled dust upon their heads towards heaven

Ye have heard of the Patience of Job and have seen the end of the Lord

WBlake inven & Sculpt

London Published as the Act directs March 8.1825 by William Blake N.s Fountain Court Strand

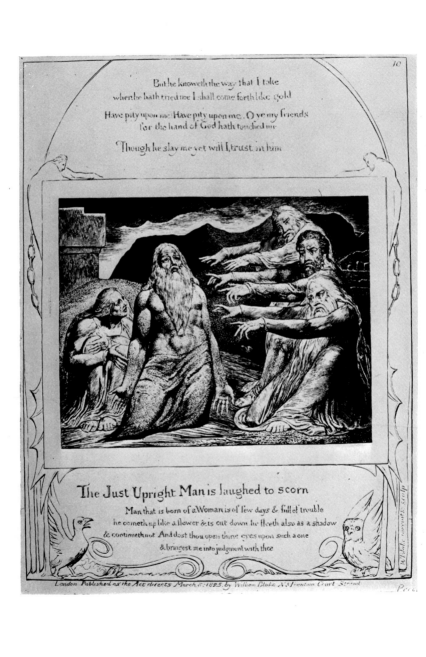

10

But he knoweth the way that I take
when he hath tried me I shall come forth like gold

Have pity upon me! Have pity upon me. O ye my friends
for the hand of God hath touched me

Though he slay me yet will I trust in him

The Just Upright Man is laughed to scorn

Man that is born of a Woman is of few days & full of trouble
he cometh up like a flower & is cut down he fleeth also as a shadow
& continueth not And dost thou open thine eyes upon such a one
& bringest me into judgment with thee

London Published as the Act directs March 8: 1825. by William Blake N.º 3 Fountain Court Strand

ards which come to him from the outside (and which he himself would
have accepted before he became ill) puts Job in the wrong. He becomes a
sinner within his religion or a rebel against it. In another context he is
either mad or bad.[4]

In his confrontation with the comforters, Job is in the same position as
the paranoid patient in hospital. If he denies being insane, his protestation
is taken as proof of his insanity. He has to admit insanity to become a
"good" patient who can later be declared sane and be discharged. Job had,
according to his comforters, to admit sin, and be contrite, in order to be
forgiven and restored to good fortune. It is a tribute to his inner strength
that, throughout all his trials, he chose to rebel.[5]

Job breaks the silence with a bitter cry of desolation and anger. The
imagery he uses is of darkness and death; light must be shut out; life should
not have begun. The imagery continues in terms of these fundamental
themes. The calamities which he has suffered have begun to be experienced as an inner anguish and distress:

> There is no peace of mind nor quiet for me;
> I chafe in torment and have no rest.
>
> (3: 26)

Eliphaz starts the first cycle of speeches with a gentle and tentative
approach to Job:

> If one ventures to speak with you, will you lose patience?
> For who could hold his tongue any longer?
> Think how once you encouraged those who faltered,
> . . .
> But now that adversity comes upon you, you lose patience;
>
> (4: 2–5)

He makes a request that Job be patient and seek from his religion some
solace in his suffering. He recalls to Job that it was he who had always
offered a helping hand to those in distress and exhorts him to seek strength

[4] The idea that the rebel is labelled "mad" or "bad" for the purposes of family
and/or society status quo has been purported by Laing and others.

[5] Hence the famous, but only partially quoted, verse:

> If he would slay me, I should not hesitate;
> I would still argue my cause to his face.
>
> (13: 15)

(See p. 71.)

from the blameless life he had led. At this point he colludes with Job in the idea of his innocence, but gently pleads with him to relinquish his claim to perfection.

Eliphaz speaks of a vision. The message was that mortal man should not try to make himself more righteous than God. This vision marks the introduction of a theme which will have a great importance in Job's treatment: the invocation of unconscious sources as having validity and authority. Job will claim his right to free association; Elihu will speak of the way in which he could no longer contain the words which come bursting forth; and the words of God, when he appears out of the whirlwind, may be a revelation audible only to Job's inner ear.

Eliphaz suggests that Job accept his lot and "not reject the discipline of the Almighty" (5: 17). If Job does this, he will be sure to be shielded from final disaster. He relies on traditional wisdom, reinforced by his certainty of an intuitive grasp of the working of the divine mind:

> We have inquired into all this, and so it is;
> this we have heard, and you may know it for the truth.
> (5: 27)

Job refutes the appeal of Eliphaz for patient acceptance of suffering. He declares that the extent of his suffering is beyond measure. He bursts out with anger against the comforters. How can they know the extent of his misfortunes? If his words are wild, it is because he is having to suffer the onslaughts of the God whose arrows find their mark in him. He does not complain without cause. He can no longer find help from within himself and neither is he getting any help from the comforters. He compares their friendship to the wadis: those rivers which run full spate and which unaccountably dry up and leave no trace for long periods. The comforters likewise are lacking in the constancy of devotion which is the due of friends. Even more, they are treacherous. Their treachery is due to their fear of contamination from illness, poverty, and distress. Many people attempt to console the sufferer more for their own peace of mind than for that of the sufferer.

Job asks them to put forward plainly where he has erred to the extent that he should be so punished. Job makes an outright challenge to them that his case be reviewed, and that an objective account of what he has done wrong be made:

> Tell me plainly, and I will listen in silence;
> show me where I have erred.
>
> (6: 24)

He exhorts them to

> Think again, let me have no more injustice;
> think again, for my integrity is in question.
>
> (6: 29)

Job's claim to perfection is his dearest possession, the only thing he has left. His sense of justice and his integrity are intricately bound up with his sense of identity:

> Do I ever give voice to injustice?
> Does my sense not warn me when my words are wild?
>
> (6: 30)

He is claiming that he knows that he is not insane. For Job, sanity means the ability to be just, and justice is part of his perfection. Perfection and sanity go hand in hand.

At the same time, Job complains bitterly of his physical ailments and persecutions from God. The more he defends his sense of justice and his sanity at this stage, the more do his feelings of persecution and the psychosomatic symptoms increase in their intensity. The tension within Job must be great at this point. The mental anguish is augmented to the degree that he tries so vigorously to maintain that pivotal self-definition of himself as perfect and upright, which we have already discussed.

It is Bildad's turn next, and he shows no diffidence in attacking Job as somebody who speaks with "the long-winded ramblings of an old man" (8: 2). Hostility answers hostility. Bildad is telling Job that he is old and confused. It is not difficult to imagine that the ambivalent relationship of the comforters with Job is made more hostile in a secret delight in his misfortune. Unlike Eliphaz, Bildad claims that Job's catastrophes were deserved, even if indirectly, through his children:

> Does the Almighty pervert justice?
> Your sons sinned against him,
> so he left them to be victims of their own iniquity.
>
> (8: 3-4)

Any comfort which Bildad can offer is conditional upon Job's acceptance
of the traditional wisdom which the comforters represent:

> Inquire now of older generations
> and consider the experience of their fathers;
> for we ourselves are of yesterday and are transient;
> our days on earth are a shadow.
> Will not they speak to you and teach you
> and pour out the wisdom of their hearts?
>
> (8: 8–10)

Job refutes the argument. He is not satisfied with the balance of
behaviour and reward, or the fairness of God's judgements. Moreover, if
he challenges God's verdict, he is sure that, when the case was argued out,
the results would be in God's favour, no matter what the merits of the
case might be:

> If a man chooses to argue with him
> God will not answer one question in a thousand.
> He is wise, he is powerful;   (9: 34)

Job goes on to ask, "What man has stubbornly resisted him and survived?" (9: 4). But Job does, nevertheless, stubbornly resist God and
survives. His final submission to God has its own meaning to be developed
later, but without Job's sustained resistance his survival and subsequent
restoration to wealth would have been worth no more than the material
possessions which he regained.

Taking this first cycle as a whole, there is a gradation of intensity in the
challenge to Job. Eliphaz had begun gently with the contemplation of the
possibility that Job was innocent. Bildad had offered the suggestion that
the sin for which the punishment was being administered might perhaps
have been that of Job's children. Zophar is the first to put the blame
squarely onto Job. He also attacks Job's personality, accusing him of
talking long-winded nonsense, and, adding for good measure, that God
was exacting from him less than his sin deserved (11:6). In completing the
first cycle of speeches of the three comforters, Zophar accuses Job outright
of having sinned and having deserved the suffering which is the result of
his sins. This is the first true confrontation—Job is directly accused of
being wicked. How else could it be, since God is always right?

> He surely knows which men are false,
> and when he sees iniquity, does he not take note of it?
> . . .
> If only you had directed your heart rightly
>
> (11: 11–13)

Job's answer to this attack shows a mastery of satirical invective:

> No doubt you are perfect men
> and absolute wisdom is yours![6]
>
> (12: 2)

He maintains his ascendancy in argument over the comforters. Full of irony, he points out that in no way do the comforters have knowledge which he does not have also (12: 3). He, too, is cognizant of traditional wisdom, and moreover he can claim the respect due to his age (12: 12). Job continues gathering strength as he claims that, not only is he the match for their combined efforts, but he is also prepared to take on God as well, and at the same time. Job's is the mastermind that can take on multiple opponents in simultaneous contests.

> But for my part I would speak with the Almighty
> and am ready to argue with God,
> while you like fools are smearing truth with your falsehoods,
> stitching a patchwork of lies, one and all.
> Ah, if you would only be silent
> and let silence be your wisdom!   (13: 3–5)

The modern psychoanalyst's self-image is of a silent participator in the therapy. It is the patient who is supposed to do the talking. And yet, whenever detailed inquiries have been made as to the actual practice, it is revealed that the psychoanalyst speaks more than he is prepared to admit. The modern patient, like Job, may resent the analyst who talks too much. After all, the situation is set up for the patient's benefit!

The cycle of speeches has offered a device for each in turn to make a contribution. But in Job's reply at the conclusion of the first cycle of speeches, he deals with them collectively. He is truly the leader of the group that came to heal him.

---

[6] Authorized Version:

> No doubt but ye are the people, and wisdom shall die with you.

Job maintains, from the depths of his suffering, that even in his dejection he has more courage than they. He has had to wrestle with his illness, the arguments and accusations of the comforters, and he is even willing to challenge God. If, in the confrontation between Job and God, the comforters intervene, they intervene falsely because they have neither a glimmer of understanding of what is happening, nor the calibre to enter into a combat with major contestants.

> He will most surely expose you
> if you take his part by falsely accusing me.
> Will not God's majesty strike you with dread,
> and terror of him overwhelm you?
> Your pompous talk is dust and ashes,
> your defences will crumble like clay.
>
> (13: 10–12)

The comforters had rested their argument on existing authorities which do not require any support, whereas Job enters into new and dangerous thoughts.

Nevertheless, it is Job who eventually wins through to security, and it is the comforters who find that their platitudinous jargon avails them nothing when they have to face Job's relentless argumentation with diminishing reserves of inner strength.

There has been a lot of talk about talking. All three comforters have justifiably accused Job of trying to out-talk them. Zophar felt that Job used words, not to develop an argument, but to wear them down ("Is your endless talk to reduce men to silence?"). Job, in reply, threatens them with the consequences of their shallow arguments and pompous talk.

It is at this point that something very important in the course of Job's illness and its treatment occurs. Job demands the right to have silence from the group and to speak whatever comes into his mind. He claims the right to free association, and he is well aware of the risk he is taking:

> Be silent, leave me to speak my mind,
> and let what may come upon me!
> I will put my neck in the noose
> and take my life in my hands.
>
> (13: 13–14)

Job's willingness to risk the thoughts, which come unbidden and uncensored, provide him with a new strength, and he shows a renewed confidence in his assertions:

> If he would slay me, I should not hesitate;
> I would still argue my cause to his face.[7]
> This at least assures my success,
> that no godless man may appear before him.
> Listen then, listen to my words,
> and give a hearing to my exposition.
> Be sure of this: once I have stated my case
> I know that I shall be acquitted.
> Who is there that can argue so forcibly with me
> that he could reduce me straightway to silence and death?
>
> (13: 15–19)

In the next chapter (14: 1–14), Job will embark on thoughts about reproduction, eternity, and about death which comes not as a punishment but as a fulfilment of sexuality. These new thoughts will form the creative part of his illness. But before this consummation, he regresses again in the need to find answers from outside sources ("Let me know my offences and my sin", 13: 23). This is part of his challenge to God, but it is to his comforters that he actually addresses his words. Even in contemporary psychotherapy, the patient is sometimes driven to find his own construction of a cure in the presence of a therapist whose mind lags behind that of the patient. Yet in such a situation, the patient from time to time turns to the therapist for answers which he feels he has the right to expect. In such a case, the treatment is a contest in which the patient learns that the answers eventually come from within his own person. Job is beginning to have this experience in this inverse therapeutic group of which in a subtle way he remains the leader.

[7] The Authorized Version translates this as:

> Though he slay me, yet will I trust in him:
> but I will maintain mine own ways before him.

The first of these two lines is one of the most widely quoted from the Book of Job as an example of supreme submission to the will of God. But the succeeding line ("but I will maintain . . .") seems to pass almost unnoticed by Bible commentators. These two lines, taken in conjunction, are a direct challenge to God, and not submission to him, and would imply Job's readiness to defend his own opinions even to the point of death.

But now, having claimed his right to free association, Job begins to ruminate about the nature of sexual reproduction.[8] Propagation of the species differs in animals and human beings from the processes in the vegetative world. In human reproduction, sex is linked with the birth of the new generation and the mortality of the progenitor. Most species of plants also have a method of reproduction through the combination of male and female elements which form seeds, and which give rise to new plants. This, too, is sexual. Many species of plants, however, are able to be reproduced in a non-sexual way by cuttings from existing parts of a mature plant. Stems, leaves, and roots can be transplanted and give rise to entirely new plants. This process may occur spontaneously (i.e. without man's aid) by runners and shoots which produce new plants a short distance away from their single parent. There is an essential difference between these two methods of reproduction. Sexual reproduction in plants, as in human beings and other animals, gives rise, through seeds, to new plants which have genetic sources in two different parent plants. Non-sexual reproduction, on the other hand, gives rise to no enrichment of the qualities of the species. It merely perpetuates (through carbon copies) the qualities of the original plant. And yet non-sexual reproduction is a kind of immortality. Sexual reproduction is associated with the genetically in-built mortality of the species (14: 5). Non-sexual reproduction grants an immortality (14: 7–9).

These thoughts are linked with the ideas of life-after-death and immortality not of the body but of a soul in which reparation could be made. Here, Job is merely hinting at ideas of immortality (14: 14). Elsewhere, he denies himself the indirect comfort of any after-life which might make amends or bring greater retribution.

Such ruminations are evidence of the growing insight which prepares Job for his cure. The fact that there is a limit to life, and that mortality is linked with sexual reproduction, and that reproduction gives rise to a new generation, brings Job out of the depth of depression which recognized no past, present, or future. The death which is associated with depression is not final as long as human beings have heirs and successors. It is a paradox that sexual reproduction, and death, provide a means by

---

[8] It might have delighted Freud if it had been pointed out to him that the first new theme which Job entered into after claiming the right to free association, was reproduction.

which man can be concerned with a future which he will not personally know. Job now accepts death, but he no longer completely abandons himself to it, for he shows concern for future generations:

> His sons rise to honour, and he sees nothing of it;
> they sink into obscurity, and he knows it not.
>
> (14: 21)

Although here he is recognizing limits to man's knowledge of the future, he is also giving expression to a very human desire to know what it might be.

The second cycle of speeches begins at this point. Eliphaz has his second chance and begins with the ritual abuse that each comforter in turn heaps upon Job, and he upon them.

> Would a man of sense give vent to such foolish notions
> and answer with a bellyful of wind?
> Would he bandy useless words
> and arguments so unprofitable?
>
> (15: 2–3)

At the same time Eliphaz finds an excuse for Job's outpourings and rescues him from the duty of having to answer them. In the modern idiom, when one member of a family is unaccountably vituperative to others, it is often said by the family doctor, "It is his illness that is speaking, not his own thoughts." Eliphaz is saying, "It is not really Job but his iniquity that is speaking." And one must recall the fact that one of the most unjust ways of answering the just complaints of a psychiatric patient is to say, "You are not yourself today." It is also one of the unfair practices of a parent to a child who appears to be naughty, "That is not my little Johnnie who is doing that." This practice is an exact replica of the situation which the comforters bring to Job. They have an idealized image (at times) of the former Job, and their therapeutic aim is to restore him to a personality which fits that image. Job himself might have accepted that aim in the earlier stages when, in reaction to the calamities, he said nothing unseemly. The Epilogue goes some way towards accepting cure at this level. But yet there is ample evidence throughout the narrative of a Job whose personality had qualities which the original Job could never have acknowledged.

Eliphaz now in his turn claims silence from Job ("I will tell you, if only you will listen" (15:17), and again appeals to the traditional wisdom of the founding fathers for answers to Job's arguments:

> (what has been handed down by wise men
> and was not concealed from them by their fathers;
> to them alone the land was given,
> and no foreigner settled among them):
>
> (15: 18–19)

The justification of the purity of the message is the purity of the race. Eliphaz is trying to denigrate whatever wisdom Job might have come to on his own account. He calls upon Job to acknowledge the pure message of a pure race, as Job himself would have done before his illness. This message is again basically that of an exact balance of justice: goodness is rewarded and evil punished in kind.

Eliphaz, ever the most ready to find some excuse for Job, suggests that the foreigners in their midst have been the incitement for Job's heterodoxy. It would seem that throughout the ages the alien immigrant is made the scapegoat for unwelcome beliefs which threaten orthodox and traditional practice. The Soncino publication commentary has this to say on this passage:

> Eliphaz claims that the tradition he represents is pure and unadulterated, and has not been contaminated by contact with foreign elements. He hints that the foreigners in their midst are responsible for Job's heretical opinions.[9]

In the later Biblical days there was constant fear of contamination by Hellenic ideas. The Soncino commentators, amongst other scholarly works on Job, show that some Hellenistic and Babylonian ideas can be found in the Book of Job. External philosophical systems were seen as a threat to Hebrew orthodoxy. Eliphaz claims that the purity of tradition has to be preserved at all costs and without regard to any pain which the acceptance of austere doctrines might involve.[10]

Eliphaz lists the horrors which befall a man who has forsaken the traditional Hebrew God. Not only can they be contaminated by ideas of the foreigner, they have also to defend themselves against his physical attack. The message is the necessity to keep one's self pure and to defend

---

[9] Soncino Version, *op. cit.*, p. 76.
[10] A contrasting message can be inferred from the Book of Ruth.

one's possessions and one's faith. The man who opens himself up to ideas other than the traditional ones has, in Eliphaz's view,

> . . . lifted his hand against God
> and is pitting himself against the Almighty,
> charging him head down,
> with the full weight of his bossed shield.
>
> (15: 25–26)

In challenging God, Job is going against tradition, and this is a perilous activity. Rebels and pioneers are vulnerable to criticism and to attacks from their own community. As a prophet, Eliphaz is on safe ground for he foretells, as the fate of the rebel against religious authority, the events which have already overtaken Job. He describes how the house of such a person is demolished, wealth destroyed, and how such an individual loses his progeny:

> and he will strike no root in the earth;
> scorching heat will shrivel his shoots,
>
> (15: 29–30)

He goes on to state that "the godless, one and all, are barren . . . and the child of their womb is deceit" (15: 34–35). He is here referring to Job's loss of children and possessions, and he is taking up the reproductive imagery which Job had previously employed. He is telling Job that his posterity has been destroyed by his wickedness and sin. Job's metaphors on reproduction were prolific in meaning: image followed image. But Eliphaz returns to the rigid doctrine in which all the variations are on the same theme.

When Eliphaz had appealed to tradition, he had been referring to the wisdom within the tradition. His defences have been weakened from prolonged argument with Job. It is to tradition *per se* that he now appeals, and not to the rationality which can be the product of wisdom. He has become more rigid and more defensive about the message which he is conveying. It would almost seem that Eliphaz and his colleagues were becoming increasingly more anxious in pace with Job's recovery. Their inability to convince Job of the rightness of their traditional case must have eroded their own faith. The dogma is more strongly asserted (15: 33–35) in the frantic efforts which precede their final exhaustion.

There is a pattern emerging here which all the comforters follow: accusation against Job, clarification of the accusation, and prediction of disaster in the future. This is followed by Job's denial, counter-accusation, and refutation of their conclusion.

Job's answer to Eliphaz is that he could be a better comforter than he:

> If you and I were to change places,
> I could talk like you;
> how I could harangue you
> and wag my head at you!
> But no, I would speak words of encouragement,
> and then my condolences would flow in streams.
>
> (16: 4–5)

Job in fact has claimed that he would be a better prophet (13: 10–11), a better teacher (12: 3), a better rhetorician (19: 23), and a better therapist ("ye are all physicians of no value", Authorized Version, 13: 4). Having successfully reversed the accustomed roles of dominance in the situation of mourner and comforter, he goes on to accuse them of conspiracy (16: 9–10). These paranoid thoughts come in the wake of the comforters' dismissal of his new insights as they once more retreat to the shelter of the wisdom of tradition. The comforters deny the validity of the truth which Job feels he has constructed out of his own experience and which is emerging from the free association of thoughts at the borderland of the unconscious.

The comforters do not allow Job to experiment with his new ideas. When everything that Job proposes is dismissed outright, anger follows frustration and persecutory thoughts follow the anger. Had Job been dependent exclusively upon their approval, this situation might have confirmed and established Job in his mental disorder. To the extent that insanity is a state of disjunction where one is insane and others sane by popular consent, [11] Job was indeed in a perilous situation. Job's behaviour included all the elements which are present in paranoid schizophrenia; but he had maintained his integrity and had consistently—even if precariously—held on to his sanity. How exasperating it must have been for the comforters to find that even in his degradation and suffering, Job was able to regain his old ascendancy. It would have been natural for them collectively to have taken the dominant position for granted. How resent-

[11] R. D. Laing, *The Divided Self, op. cit.*, p. 37 (see Chapter 3).

ful they must have felt against Job's manner which was that of a superior to inferiors:

> What do you mean by treating us as cattle?
> Are we nothing but brute beasts to you?
>
> (18: 3)

The comforters had now come to regard Job as incurably obstinate, and Job was seeing them as being in persecutory conspiracy.

The comforters call on Job to admit his guilt. He must repent for past sins. The evidence of his wrongdoing is the punishment which he is receiving. He must admit the guilt in order to be forgiven. This is an attempt to trap Job. Job is offered no way of claiming that his past behaviour has been good and that he was being punished without cause. The comforters add another argument: to be mortal is inevitably to be sinful ("What is frail man that he should be innocent, or any child of woman that he should be justified?" 15: 14). During birth, the child has the experience of moving through the sexual passages of a woman. By this reasoning, Job must have sinned, even though he did not know it. But repentance on these terms must be ineffectual, as how can repentance be genuine, and lead to alteration in conduct (becoming good), without a recital of the specific details of the sins which have been committed (the badness)?

These themes, arising in what we have been claiming is the therapeutic situation, are the essence of what has already been referred to as the "double bind". This paradox, where the therapeutic procedures are potentially pathogenic, is not out of keeping with some modern views of the part played by the authoritative figures in society, including therapists, in the process of establishing and labelling of insanity in some chosen member. The double bind is described typically in the relationship of a mother and child where the child is given ambiguous messages to which any response is wrong. The child is in a "no win" position, and it would seem that his only way of not being wrong is to be completely inactive, i.e. to give no response at all.

In a simple way, double bind messages are everybody's experience. A child may be repeatedly told by his parents that they expect him to get good positions in school examinations, and then criticize him for being a bookworm. They may issue dire warnings to an adolescent girl about the dangers of sexual contacts, and then ask her why she does not have as many boyfriends as other girls. Bateson's own example is of a

> . . . young man who had fairly well recovered from an acute schizophrenic episode [and who] was visited in the hospital by his mother. He was glad to see her and impulsively put his arm around her shoulders, whereupon she stiffened. He withdrew his arm and she asked, "Don't you love me any more?" He then blushed, and she said, "Dear, you must not be so easily embarrassed and afraid of your feelings."[12]

The components of the double bind situation have been described as including

> a framework of relationships with significant others; the need to discriminate correctly (given the importance of the dependence-independence conflict); the impossibility of leaving the field (given the dependency inherent in childhood); the impossibility of asking for clarification; and finally a message that contains an injunction regarding a concrete fact and a second injunction regarding this class of facts that contradict the first.[13]

The concept of the double bind has been amplified by Virginia Satir.[14] She points out that the double bind can not be operative unless the victim is dependent for approval on the individual who gives the ambiguous message. An individual receiving such an ambiguous message may extricate himself from the double bind, and its pathogenic consequences merely by asking for a clarification of the message. The hostile criticism given with a gentle smile is intended to imply, "I am not really being hostile." If hostility is positively denied, the recipient can say, "But it didn't sound like that to me."

Kafka[15] offers a critical evaluation of the double bind theory by stating that ambiguity is an essential requisite for normal development. He acknowledges that over-exposure to paradoxical communications is poten-

[12] G. Bateson, D. D. Jackson, J. Haley *et al.*, *op. cit.*

[13] Sluzki and Veron, "The double bind as a universal pathogenic situation", *Family Process*, **10** (Dec. 1971), pp. 397–410 as abstracted by Elizabeth Groff, *Digest of Neurology and Psychiatry*, **39** (Dec. 1971), p. 439.

[14] Virginia Satir, *Conjoint Family Therapy*, rev. ed. (Calif.: Science and Behavior Books, 1967), p. 36.

[15] John S. Kafka, "Ambiguity for individuation", *Arch Gen Psychiat.* **25** (Sept. 1971).

tially pathogenic. A command which is a deliberate trap paralyses action, particularly in cases where an individual is instructed to take more initiative but is told that any action he takes is wrong. Under-exposure to ambiguous communications, on the other hand, results from a fear of paradox on the part of the parent.

In the system underlying the assumptions of the double bind theory every communication is expected to have only one meaning and every activity must be the correct one. Knowledge must be scientific and exact. Such a system does not allow for essential ambiguities in words and actions. It is assumed that every problem has a solution, if only we use the right tools and possess the right information. Anything outside what is approved is bad or mad. The choice is between accepting a narrow range of permitted thought and behaviour or, alternatively, acknowledging being delinquent or mentally ill whenever one goes beyond the scheduled boundaries.

There is a need to create a third system in which one can accept *approximate* meaning, *approximate* virtue, *approximate* satisfaction, and *approximate* justice.

It might be held that jokes are tolerated ambiguity permitting new levels of communication. They may be destructive of meaning or they may create new insights. Job did not hesitate to employ irony towards his comforters regardless of the consequences.

Job had so far separated himself from the system of thought of his comforters that he was able to challenge their formulations. Some of his irony was destructive, but he took many opportunities to turn their statements round and discover new perspectives. When the comforters used the double bind, Job appealed over their heads directly to God. When they claimed absolute truth for their own statements, he was able to formulate an opposing view. Job, no doubt, had originally succumbed to the double bind situation in the religious culture which he had shared with his friends. He escaped from the double bind through having the advantage of hearing the basic themes reformulated by the comforters in the special life of the group in which all external realities were temporarily in suspense.

It is possible to see the "comfort" which Job's three friends offered him in this light. Without their admonitions and attacks, and without the protective barrier which they had created between him and the ordinary world of everyday affairs, Job would not have experienced the stimulus to gain new insights which eventually lead to his growth and cure.

Bildad (18: 12–21) reiterates to Job the threats of obliteration of personality and of posterity, and the destruction of possessions, which is the "fate of the dwellings of evildoers" (18: 21). Bildad is making every effort to muster the forces which will make Job surrender to any guilt which may still exist within him.

Job is swayed but does not surrender. He allows himself to consider for the sake of argument that he may have been in the wrong:

> If in fact I had erred,
> the error would still be mine.
>
> (19: 4)

Job is implying that on any balance sheet he is still in credit, just as Mark Antony said of the accusation that Caesar was ambitious:

> If it were so, it was a grievous fault.
> And grievously hath Caesar answer'd it.

The formulation is one which denies guilt but which, at the same time, offers a secondary defence in case the accusation is found to have some basis. This secondary defence is that *if* it should be proved true, it would be of only minor importance. The same "if" is used delicately by Touchstone in *As You Like It*: "Your If is the only peace-maker; much virtue in If."

In Job's final statement to his comforters, he reasserts his innocence. The force of his argument (that suffering can come by chance) rests upon his ability to say, in effect, "I may have suffered, but I was not evil." This allows him to escape from the position of religious determinism (spiritual "causes" which have material "effects") and venture into the speculation that chance is a valid explanation of the sequence of some events. He can now claim to be released from the inevitability of the law of cause and effect.

At this stage Job does not yet know that he will admit the human *imperfection* of limits to knowledge and power. His initial *perfection* was moral, physical, and material, and was expressed in his behaviour, his health, and his wealth. He further claimed perfection in the validity of his counselling to those who were in an inferior condition. His knowledge was standardized and readily at hand. This capacity was the fence around his perfection, but during the responses to the comforters he became prepared to put his perfection at risk by allowing spontaneity to his words.

The progress which Job is making is interrupted from time to time by periods of regression. Bildad's tirade is powerful enough. He dwells on Job's impotence and sterility and his lack of any influence on the future. The worst fear of man is that nothing that he can do will have any effect on what comes after. This has been described by psychoanalysts as castration fear which extends beyond sex into the power to have effect on the actions of contemporaries.

Job's reply resounds with despair:

> If I cry "Murder!" no one answers;
> if I appeal for help, I get no justice.
> (19: 7)

Job has returned to his feelings of isolation and persecution, and, in fact, the comforters may have felt good reason for their attempt to subjugate their troublesome contemporary. In many a therapeutic situation, there are therapists who seem to find good reasons for keeping the patient ill. Although it is true that the paranoid patient behaves in an unduly suspicious way, and has identifiable delusions of persecution, it is important also to note once more that most of the delusions which paranoid individuals report have some foundation. The exclusion is based on reality. Lemert has pointed out that although the paranoid person reacts in a characteristic way to "others" in the social environment, it is also true that "others" react differentially to him. There is an organized and conspiratorial pattern of behaviour (in a very real sense) in which a process of exclusion develops. This, in fact, is a reciprocal relationship of the paranoid person and "others".[16]

Job and his comforters have now established such a reciprocal relationship, persecuting one another with curses and counter-curses. Job calls upon his friends to "beware of the sword that points at" them (19: 29). It will soon be their turn to know that there is a judge. Job is anticipating the point at which God will pronounce them to be in the wrong, and when, but for Job's intercession, they would have suffered in like manner.

The comforters are again drawn into the deep levels of feeling which

[16] E. M. Lemert, "Dynamics of exclusion", *op. cit.*, p. 273 (see Chapter 3).

Job exhibits. Zophar in his next contribution refers to the distress of his mind. He is being disturbed by "arguments that are a reproach to me" (20: 3), and calls upon a spirit beyond his understanding to give him the answer. He, too, is allowing himself to express thoughts which come from his inner turmoil, but the message ends as usual with an appeal to traditional wisdom and with threats to the godless (20: 5).

Zophar cannot completely refute Job's statement that the wicked may prosper (just as the righteous may suffer), but he uses the device of saying that, even if reward and punishment do not immediately follow good and evil, there will be a time in the future when the reckoning will be made out. Perhaps the balance is restored through the younger generation (21: 10).

Zophar describes Job's present state of suffering in an oblique fashion, in order to threaten Job and prove him wrong ("his well-being does not last", 20: 21).

In Job's reply, which completes the second cycle of speeches, he arrives with clear conviction at the conclusion that the fate of man is not rational.

He begins with an appeal to the comforters to hear him out:

> Listen to me, do but listen,
> and let that be the comfort you offer me.
> (21: 2)

This is a plea which has had to have been made again and again in history by those who suffer and which only in recent years has been incorporated into the techniques of psychotherapy and counselling. Freud's discovery of the value of using free association came from his spontaneous response to an interjection of a woman patient. Up to that time, Freud was given to urging, pressing, and questioning his patients in his attempts to uncover the roots of their symptoms in their early life. Ernest Jones records that

> On one historic occasion, however, the patient, Frl. Elisabeth, reproved him for interrupting her flow of thought by his questions. He took the hint, and thus made another step towards free association.[17]

Job asks for silence. He does not ask the comforters to be influenced by his words. Afterwards they may mock on (21: 3). In the Authorized

[17] Ernest Jones, *Sigmund Freud: Life and Work*, (London: Hogarth Press, 1953), Vol. 1, p. 268.

Version, the implication is that his words are not to them; in fact, they are addressed not to man but to God. The New English Version reads, "May not I too voice my thoughts?" (21: 4).

Job is reaching down to an inner spirit which is the unconscious. He is aware of the danger of this undertaking, which Reich has called "the journey into the dark continent";

> When I stop to think, I am filled with horror,
> and my whole body is convulsed.   (21: 6)

These phrases are not merely the heroics of drama. They are the reality of the experience of emotion which comes at moments of religious conversion or during the uncovering of hidden depths of the mind. Essential as the comforters are as stimulators of and witnesses to the process, Job is now addressing his own self, and is facing the necessary inner turmoil.

The themes derive from his confidence in his own observations and his experience that natural disasters encompass the good and the wicked alike. Even more, in these circumstances, it is often the wicked and the unscrupulous who escape (21: 29–30). He once again challenges the comforters' use of the argument that his misfortune is proof of his iniquity. His superiority is now such that, not only is he in control of his own thoughts, but also can he anticipate what the comforters might say in answer:

> I know well what you are thinking
> and the arguments you are marshalling against me;
> (21: 27)

In the subsequent argument, Job completely demolishes the idea of retributive justice. Meanwhile, he is approaching a somewhat unaccustomed humility:

> Can any man teach God,
> God who judges even those in heaven above?
> (21: 22)

Perhaps this acknowledgement of the inscrutability of God was intended as an argument to the comforters that God was not bound by *their* system, but, by the same token, Job himself has had to acknowledge that there ocu1d be knowledge beyond any that he himself had access to. It may be that he was caught by his own argument and had to accept the consequences.

If we return to the dramatic idiom, the third cycle of speeches resembles the anticlimax which precedes the dénouement in many plays. Eliphaz makes the opening speech, and it appears that he is influenced by Job's latest point. He seems to be prepared to submit to the view that the goodness of man can add nothing to God (22: 3). He develops it a little further. Job had stated that the wicked man often goes unpunished. Eliphaz adds that the good man is no benefit to God. Being perfect, God has nothing to gain from the perfection of man.

Eliphaz, however, returns to the previous generalizations on wickedness and retribution. He then goes further and asserts that Job was totally bad (22: 4). Job, on his part, continually claims that he had always acted with perfect goodness. Neither seemed to be ready to consider that some degree of goodness could be mixed with a proportion of badness. Within the retributive system which Eliphaz was employing, it would have been enough if Job had committed only one sin. A single flaw in his perfection would have justified his suffering, and if perfection is not absolute, there is no reason why suffering should not be infinite. Repentance would be required for the lapse from complete virtue, and to come to terms with God would be the way to mend his fortune (22: 21). Eliphaz goes on to promise Job a return to God's favour, thus passing from abstract argument to a concrete promise such as one would use in coaxing a child. He uses phrases such as "mend your ways", "come to terms", "come back in true sincerity", asserting that Job would be delivered if his hands were clean (22: 30).

Job begins his reply to Eliphaz with the statement, "My thoughts today are resentful" (23: 2).[18] Within the framework of traditional psycho-

---

[18] This prompts the speculation that the cycle of speeches had continued over a period of many days. Amongst the many contemporary innovations in psychotherapy there is a procedure described as "marathon group therapy". It is a variation of psychotherapy in which the intensity and urgency of the experience is enhanced by seclusion from ordinary tasks of living over several days. Stoller states that the benefit depends more upon the participants' experience of one another than in the didactic qualities of their contributions. F. H. Stoller, "A stage for trust", in A. Burton (Ed.), *Encounter: The Theory and Practice of Encounter Groups* (San Francisco: Jossey-Bass, 1969).

therapy, the opening words of this speech somewhat resemble the beginning of a psychotherapeutic session. The words are a link between the present and the previous sessions, and they carry a hint of contemplation of future progress.

The successive and recurring sessions devoted to free associations of thought found a mention, long before the invention of psychoanalysis, in Shakespeare's Sonnet XXX. Every single line of this sonnet can be said to epitomize some cry that came straight from the heart of Job.

> When to the sessions of sweet silent thought
> I summon up remembrance of things past,
> I sigh the lack of many a thing I sought,
> And with old woes new wail my dear times' waste:
> Then can I drown an eye, unus'd to flow,
> For precious friends hid in death's dateless night,
> And weep afresh love's long since cancell'd woe,
> And moan the expense of many a vanish'd sight:
> Then can I grieve at grievances foregone,
> And heavily from woe to woe tell o'er
> The sad account of fore-bemoaned moan,
> Which I new pay as if not paid before.
>> But if the while I think on thee, dear friend,
>> All losses are restor'd and sorrows end.

We have quoted it in full because, by now, the reader, too, is becoming prepared for the relief that Job is about to experience. "My thoughts today are resentful; yesterday they were different; tomorrow they will have changed again."

Job now refers to his sufferings in a more contemplative mood. He is not so bitter or so angry as before, but in asking to come before the Almighty he ruminates on the arguments he might use (23: 4). He toys with the idea that now he would understand the words which God would speak to him (23: 6), and is prepared to envisage a God who would neither bring a charge against him nor use the full extent of his power over him. This God, however, is elusive:

> If I go forward, he is not there;
> if backward, I cannot find him;
> when I turn left, I do not descry him;
> I face right, but I see him not.
>
> (23: 8–9)

Job cannot pin God down, neither in place nor in time:

> The day of reckoning is no secret to the Almighty,
> though those who know him have no hint of its date.
>
> (24: 2)

It is as if the sessions of the court are fixed but no one is allowed to know when the hearings will take place.

There is something youthful in Job's urge to go beyond the comforters and take his case to God in order to put forward his grievance about the injustice and suffering in the world. He would now state his case, set out his arguments, and learn the answer that God would give (23: 3–5). In this urgency, he forgets what he has already learnt: that goodness and badness do not receive proportionate reward. He is addressing a personal and paternal God with the faith and confidence that he would "never bring a charge against me" (23: 6), and (inconsistently) he adds, "and I shall win from my judge an absolute discharge" (23: 7). At this stage, Job's God is benevolent and understanding. If he had appeared harsh, it was because the comforters had carried the wrong messages between Job and God.

Two contentions follow. First, Job claims that he has never transgressed and that his feet had kept to the path which God had set him (13: 11). The second is that God is beyond man's control (23: 13). The failure of his obsessional practices gives proof that Job himself has no control over God's decisions. And now Job is beginning to lose his need for these obsessional activities.

This relinquishing of his desire to control God is the occasion of a new fear, which is no longer that of punishment for sin. It is the awe of a more mysterious God who makes him faint-hearted (23: 15–16). At this new level, Job conquers his fear, and he is able to say:

> yet I am not reduced to silence by the darkness
> nor by the mystery which hides him.
>
> (23: 17)

If Job's presumption in seeking to gain answers from God concerning the nature of human suffering is pathological, then the healthy aspect which has remained within him is the intellectual purity of his struggle to find some answers himself to this question. Of even more importance, he is becoming content to leave something still wrapped in mystery.

Job had discovered that, perfect though he be in his own eyes, God still had the power to do what he wished. God cannot be governed and constrained by the way in which men carry out God's rules. If there is no rationality in God's actions, and no absolute justice, there is in man no absolute perfection other than the good which men try to accomplish for its own sake. Although Job will maintain his belief in his perfection, we can assume that from now on he will remain virtuous for virtue's sake, and not for the sake of any reward.

It is at this point that Job can relinquish his perfection in absolute form. Living processes can be understood by scientific laws which are a convenient approximation to what really happens. The reality is more complex than scientific laws can encompass. Modern physics has had to recapitulate Job's progress from determinacy to indeterminacy. In the nineteenth century it was taken for granted that all scientific laws could be framed in causal form. Difficulties began to occur when the minute particles of matter were shown to have direction which by its nature could not be predicted. A formal principle was put forward by Heisenberg in 1927 under the name of "the principle of uncertainty". He showed that every description of nature contains some essential uncertainty and that this uncertainty was a positive quality rather than a deficiency in knowledge about the events which are being described. The same principle had already been recognized in literature and the arts by poets who deliberately permitted themselves the use of stream of consciousness, and by surrealist and symbolist artists who were not appalled by inconsistencies in perception.

Psychology has made its recent progress in two stages in the same manner as physics. When determinacy was introduced into mental life, the concept of "motive" was made the equivalent of "cause". Behaviour was seen as the effect. With this in mind, even the dynamic schools of psychology were made mechanistic. It was a further stage of progress to recognize that although events could be traced back to causes, the future could not be predicted. At any one stage, a number of alternative courses were possible.[19]

In a similar manner, moral laws must assume an indeterminacy which is lacking in the perfection which had previously been attributed to God. The scientist has not escaped attributing such perfection, if not to God,

[19] Sigmund Freud, "The psychogenesis of a case of homosexuality in a woman" (1920), *Standard Edition*, Vol XVIII (Hogarth Press, 1957) p. 167.

then to a grand design in nature which is the final cause of every happening.

This is an idea which Eliphaz had approached when he spoke of the course of wicked men:

> Yet it was he [God] that filled their houses with good things,
> although their purposes and his were very different.
>
> (22: 18)

but he was unable to carry it to its logical conclusion. This is the first idea Job was able to take from a comforter and develop, instead of sweeping it away with counter arguments. This also is the first step which Job has taken towards accepting a position as an equal to some other human being rather than as a superior, parent, teacher, or religious authority. In a group, it would be his first step towards membership as a participant, rather than as the leader.

Bildad's final speech is the shortest of the Book, comprising no more than six verses. The shortness of this speech, and the fact that the third comforter, Zophar, does not even take his turn, is a sign that the group which has formed around Job has almost exhausted its store of ready argument and can no longer marshall the energies needed to cope with Job's new observations.

Bildad, meanwhile, recovers sufficiently to offer a change of metaphor. He evokes a complete contrast between man and God. God has authority and power

> Authority and awe rest with him
> who has established peace in his realm on high.
> His squadrons are without number;
> at whom will they not spring from ambush?
>
> (25: 2–3)

The notion is that there is peace in heaven because there are enough defences to assure security. Perhaps Bildad wished that he and his colleagues had sufficient strength to master Job's attack so that they could regain their sense of security. But man is different, and his weakness rests on the sexuality which denies him the plea of "not guilty":

> How then can a man be justified in God's sight,
> or one born of woman be innocent?   (25: 4)

In a psychological sense, Bildad utilizes the guilt which is associated with sexual reproduction and personal mortality in order to contrast the idea of God's purity which is connected with immortality. In so far as man is a sexual being, he is necessarily less than perfect. Job should abrogate his claim to perfection. It is interesting to note the difference between Job's and Bildad's approach to sexuality. When Job had ruminaetd on sexuality, his thoughts led him towards speculations on the nature of mortality and immortality. With Bildad, the emphasis is on guilt.

Bildad ends his own arguments—and, collectively, those of the group of comforters—by comparing man to a maggot, as lowly in relation to God as the moon and stars are in relation to the sun. Bildad is not personalizing Job's guilt here, but is making a general statement about man. In this sense, it could be healing to Job, because Bildad is now pinpointing Job's position merely as a representative of the condition of man. He offers a generality and is asking the assembled group to look upon Job's plight in a new perspective. Job has been claiming perfection, but any perfection which a man may claim must be of a dimness which is almost undiscernible in comparison with the perfection of God. It is the darkness visible.

The speech of Bildad has ended the contribution of the comforters. They are now exhausted and reduced to silence.

The trends which we have drawn out of the narrative so far have been in the progression in Job's feelings and experiences of himself. He had shared in the traditional religious view, and had then gone on to challenge God within the terms of this tradition. The comforters dealt gently with him at first, believing him to be innocent, but, by his refusal to accept his suffering as the judgement of a righteous God, he was challenging *their* faith and *their* tradition. They answered him with vituperation. Job, who had been depressed, and then angry, now began to make accusations of being persecuted.

The experience of depression, and its gradual recovery, provided Job with a personal model of the goodness and badness which had existed within himself. Later, this enabled him to see goodness in the external world. Conversely, we can say that his final perception of the goodness of the external world enabled him to reactivate his perceptions of the goodness within himself. This new perception of the self and of the outside world was occasioned by the group experience. Job himself had sought nothing more than a return to his previous state of health in which his experience of wholeness rested on his traditional beliefs. The comforters reiterated those beliefs as if spoken by his former self. This provided the therapeutic situation in which he recapitulated his ideas, poured out his woes, and discovered the falsity of the old comfort. Within the illness was a creative factor which enabled Job to turn the transactions with the comforters into a therapeutic process which we shall study further.

CHAPTER 6

Battle with Perfection

BEFORE a person can search out a cure for a psychiatric condition, it is necessary for him to acknowledge that he is ill. There is a corollary, in that society also has to acknowledge the existence of psychiatric illness in general before psychotherapy becomes part of its resources.[1] In a comparable manner, it could be said that one can gain communion with the Deity only by acknowledging the existence of human sinfulness.

Job steadfastly refused to admit that he had sinned; and at the same time, however much he suffered, he maintained his belief in his sanity. Job's faith in his perfection both sustained him during his suffering and denied him release from it.

It will be our theme in this and the following chapter that it was through the abandonment of his perfection that Job finally achieved a higher level of spiritual understanding and, at the same time, came through his turmoil into a new level of mental stability.

We must recognize that within the contemporary values, Job had a right to insist on the perfection of his behaviour and on the integrity of his

---

[1] Jules Coleman comments:

> A member of a particular society can regard himself as having an emotional illness—for which proper treatment is psychotherapy—only if his society recognises the existence of such illness and sanctions psychotherapy as the appropriate treatment for them.

Jules Coleman, "Social factors influencing the development and containment of psychiatric symptoms", in T. J. Scheff (Ed.), *Mental Illness and Social Processes*, p. 170.

mental state. Nevertheless, in a modern setting, his inner turmoil would have merited a clinical label.[2] Cure[3] was only achieved when finally he released himself from his claim to perfection.

Granted that it is appropriate to find a clinical label, the choice of which label, and of when and how it should be applied, poses problems in regard to present-day professional definitions. Many observers of human behaviour, who study the way in which people become categorized as deviant, completely deny the concept of mental illness. They reject the psychiatric diagnosis of disordered behaviour lest those who become thus categorized are the worse off for the label.[4] In this they are taking an extreme view which is opposite to that of therapists who maintain the professional axiom that there is no such thing as badness or sin. Undesirable behaviour for them is in itself the evidence of sickness. In both these opposing approaches, the aim is to avoid injustice or disadvantage consequent upon the particular label which happens to be in common use. Job fought against the attribution of either label in the belief that he would be misrepresented or misjudged.

Only too often does it happen that treatment and religious consolation alike are given in a patronizing or even degrading way which vitiates the benefit.[5] And yet those who seek to withhold psychiatric treatment (or absolution) on the grounds that it is first necessary to give a label are also denying to human beings the reality of their inner suffering and the benefit of treatment that could be to their advantage.

[2] *Viz.* our discussion in Chapter 3.

[3] The *O.E.D.* gives the following amongst the definitions of the word "cure":

I. Care, charge, spiritual charge. . . . 4a. The spiritual charge or oversight of parishioners or lay people; the office or function of a curate. Commonly in phrase "cure of souls". . . .

II. Medical or remedial treatment. . . . 7. A means of healing; a remedy; a thing, action, or process that restores health.

[4] T. S. Szasz, *The Manufacture of Madness* (London: Routledge & Kegan Paul, 1971). Szasz is prominent amongst those writers who have examined the imperfections of psychiatric institutions and compare the activities of psychiatrists with their patients with political persecutions of the present day and the witch hunts of mediaeval times.

[5] For no man of such a salve can speak

That heals the wound and cures not the disgrace;

(Shakespeare, Sonnet XXXIV)

The identification of imperfections can offer the advantage of access to the help which relieves the condition denoted by the label. Thus, if a person can acknowledge that he is mentally ill, and, as a result of that acknowledgement, can receive effective treatment, then he does not suffer from the label but gains from it. The label becomes his entitlement to relief which he would not otherwise receive.

Elihu speaks of the "price of his release" when referring to the meaning of Job's suffering. The price of release from suffering is paid for in the way in which help is solicited, received, and understood, and is something which is experienced through the different stages of human life from infancy to old age.

In times of need, people seek the availability of their fellow creatures. Infancy is a time when the need is perpetual, and yet the infant's cry can be perceived as an appeal for help or as an intrusion. There is a modern tendency to regard the infant's cry as something extraneous or illegitimate. It has been said that this tendency for mothers to resist paying attention to the infant's cry is due to a general fear, first that the child will be spoiled, and, secondly, that the mother will be exploited. Of course, mothers still continue to pay attention to certain of their infant's cries, and they have a device by which they permit themselves to give help: the legitimization resides in the "serious" nature of the demand, with the mother as judge of its seriousness.

There are various ways in which people who suffer external loss or inner distress can make their needs known to other people, and there are a corresponding number of ways in which a response can be made. They all involve labelling. The professions respond if the cry is made within the terms which fit the image of that profession.

One has to know what a doctor will treat in order to get the doctor's help. The labels which are given, and which have to be accepted by the patient as part of the price of receiving help, are the diagnostic categories.

In a religious setting, it is often conceived that God's help can be gained by the confession of "sinfulness", "unworthiness", or "simplicity" (all being labels).

When Job suffered his material losses and his bereavements, he experienced coincidentally a breach in his physical perfection. His losses made him into a mourner, and this was the label which gave him the right to the comfort of his friends. But, as his suffering went on, and as the effectiveness of the consolation appeared to be insufficient, new labels had to be provided. The comforters then decided that his suffering was continuing because Job was a sinner (a "wicked man"). Job refused to accept this new label.

Had he lived in another age, he might, as an alternative, have sought medical help on a physical or psychiatric level. His symptoms would have had to fit an image that would already be present in the medical mind. The structuring of the complaint along the lines of diagnosis, prognosis, and treatment would be done by the professional person within the terms of the knowledge and under the system of labelling which the profession possessed.

We, at this far distance, have already fitted Job's symptoms into various psychiatric configurations. We could also trace, in his subsequent recovery, similarities to some of the modern processes of psychotherapy. But we can turn from this more specific professionalized form of presentation of symptoms and prescription of treatment to a more general concept of the way in which one human being helps another in a manner comparable with that of a mother comforting her child.

Each individual, in the light of previous experiences of receiving help from another person, may build up for himself an image of normality, an image of departure from normality, and an image of what is necessary in order to regain normality. The experience of falling ill, acknowledging it, putting oneself out of circulation, and receiving such help as comes, depends upon a pattern already laid down.

Many people become able to construct their own cures in the image of what was done for them in their infancy. One has to learn from the affection in the mother's eyes how to recognize when one is entitled to be ill and when it is "serious". Those people who have never been permitted to be ill, or who never had anything seriously wrong, are not able to "break down" until the damage is so severe that it may be irreversible.

In some cases the intervention of an outside person is necessary before illness can be acknowledged, and permission has to be granted before it can take its shape. Recovery, too, may depend upon the intervention of the outside person.

In other cases the self-image includes the capacity to fall ill and the personality has within it a store of potential recovery which is an inner confidence in the continuity of their lives. There is a central core which endures unchanged throughout the various experiences of a harmful nature. Job had preserved some of this inner confidence, and this was a personal contribution to the therapeutic process.

In Job's case the external intervention came from the comforters, whose transactions and communications drew Job into a therapeutic group. For the final process of cure, we shall have to turn to the developments in Job's personality which follow upon his inner contemplation.

At the completion of the debate with the three comforters, Job commands his audience with an uninterrupted speech which fills six chapters of the Bible text (26–31), the last four being designated (New English Version) as "Job's final survey of his case". At the end of his review, it is then Job's turn to remain silent while he listens without interruption to the subsequent intervention of Elihu, whose speech also requires six chapters (32–37). In the final phase, God is made to give an answer to Job (38–41). All that remains to be told is in the six verses of Job's concluding remarks and the Epilogue.

To resume, when Job was first stricken, he separated himself from the remainder of his family.[6] He sat apart among the ashes. Therapy began when the comforters arrived and he was no longer alone. The comforters provided the human context which we have called the therapeutic situation. The actual cure will come from within Job himself, but, without the comforters it would not have been begun.

Job and the three comforters had reached deadlock in their arguments, but certain changes in Job had already occurred. He had begun in dejection, wishing that he had never been born. In the course of the exchanges, Job began to venture new thoughts and gained a renewed confidence in the truth of his own observations, in comparison with the accepted generalizations to which the comforters had given voice in the name of traditional wisdom. He could no longer uphold the idea that reward was related in exact proportion to moral worth. He had appealed to the justice of a just God, but had become aware that God cannot be regulated by the moral laws by which men seek to rule their own lives.

His physical symptoms were at their worst when, at the beginning of

---

[6] This includes not only his wife but also, as the Septuagint Bible shows (19:17), his concubines and their children.

the narrative, he "did not utter one sinful word". Once he began to express his anger, to experience his depression, and to give utterance to his feelings of persecution, the physical component of his symptoms seemed to subside. To the extent that they still persisted, they had become of less importance to him than his turbulent thoughts.

In most respects Job remained the leader of the group that formed around him. The comforters were incapable of bettering—or even battering—him in argument. Finally they were left exhausted and silent.

What does not yet subside is Job's continued claim to innocence and perfection, and his questioning of why he was made to undergo his suffering if, indeed, he had not sinned. He remains steadfast in his conviction that in a lawful confrontation with God, he would be able to put his case in such a way that he would be found "not guilty", and that his punishments would be seen to have been administered without cause.

In Job's first words after the conclusion of the utterances of the comforters, there is a feeling that something more in Job's personal development still remains to be accomplished. He declares, yet again, "God has denied me justice" (27: 2); he is still filled with bitterness (27: 2); he is adamant that "till death, I will not abandon my claim to innocence. . . . I will not change" (27: 5-6). Yet there is an inconsistency. In the same chapter (27: 11-23), he describes how God deals with the wicked man, and his description of the wicked man's fate is similar to his own plight:

> He may have many sons, but they will fall by the sword,
> . . .
> He may lie down rich one day, but never again;
> he opens his eyes and all is gone.
> Disaster overtakes him like a flood,
> and a storm snatches him away in the night;
> the east wind lifts him up and he is gone;
> it whirls him far from home;
> it flings itself on him without mercy,
> and he is battered and buffeted by its force;
> it snaps its fingers at him
> and whistles over him wherever he may be.   (27: 14-23)

So the dilemma still remains. On the one hand, Job remains confident in his innocence. On the other, he describes with only too much insight the fate of the wicked man. Within the argument which Job continues inside himself, he has arrived at as much of a deadlock as that in which he and the comforters together had found themselves.[7]

A new viewpoint (chapter 26) offers a way out. Instead of trying to equate man's moral nature with his experience of a moral God, he allows himself to recognize the infinite power of God as reflected in the power of nature, over which man has no control. Job now links his idea of God with the power which man perceives in nature:

> God spreads the canopy of the sky over chaos
> and suspends earth in the void.
> He keeps the waters penned in dense cloud-masses,
> and the clouds do not burst open under their weight.
> He covers the face of the full moon,
> unrolling his clouds across it.
> He has fixed the horizon on the surface of the waters
> at the farthest limit of light and darkness.   (26: 7–10)

Job has been following a train of thought in regard to man's position *vis-à-vis* nature and the idea of God. As long as God is a personal judge of man, the forces of nature merely provide the material resources for God's aims. Job's argument with God from the position of perfection would have entitled him to a share in the ruling of nature. This was within a system of moral determinism where to obey the rules could guarantee the desired effects. This resembles present-day physical determinism, where the rules are called scientific laws. In either case, the essence is man's claim to power over the universe. Its practical expression is the effort to control his own

[7] The Soncino Version (*op. cit.*, p. 137) supplies a different interpretation of this passage. The implication is that Job is making an ironical statement following directly on the phrase, "why then do you talk such empty nonsense?" (27: 12). The passage, "this is the lot prescribed by God for the wicked", would be an example of the nonsense which the comforters have spoken.

"Verses 11–23 have long been a source of difficulty to the commentators involving, as it seems, a contradiction and reversal of Job's previous position that an evil fate does *not* overtake the wicked. They who maintain the integrity of the text explain the passage as the triumph, if only temporary, of Job's deep-rooted faith over the bitter indictment of God's injustice as experienced by him. Alternatively, it has been explained as Job's ironical presentation of his friends' doctrine, as in xxiv. It should be remembered that ancient writers used no punctuation marks, and the change of speaker was indicated by the inflection of the reader's voice."

fate. At every stage of civilization, there is a central problem of adjusting to the extensions of the claim to omnipotent power over human thoughts, human behaviour, and over the physical environment.

Job is now beginning to glimpse forces of nature outside the control and comprehension of man. He relinquishes the possibility of acquiring the power which he now attributes to God:

> These are but the fringe of his power;
> and how faint the whisper that we hear of him!
> (Who could fathom the thunder of his might?)
> (26: 14)

In his imagination, Job had stretched himself to equality with God and this had led him to the false position of being a judge to God. Now he allows himself to approach the idea of human limitations, i.e. to the idea of his own humanity.

Throughout the Bible passages at this stage, the theme of boundaries and limitations is repeated. This also is one of the themes which we can use to describe phases of human development from infancy to maturity. Early infancy, with the powerlessness of immaturity, has also the lack of boundaries which are inherent in phantasies of omnipotence. In the psychoanalytical formulation of the Oedipal situation (which comes later), the essential feature is the child's image of himself as the equal and rival of the powerful parent. Maturity (much later still) can only be achieved after a number of shifts in the relative balance of power between the self and others. Maturity is an acceptance of boundaries and limitations. The individual passes from the phantasy of complete power to the more truly powerful reality of limited strength. In his growing maturity, Job derives this concept of relative power from his idea of nature, and of God.

Job, however, reverts to his argumentative contest with God (chapter 27). His protestation of his innocence becomes stronger and firmer. Whatever God's power might be, Job claims to have received its spirit which would survive in him to his last breath. It is this breath of God which gives him the right to challenge God. And why not, if man is made in God's image?

God has denied Job justice within Job's own understanding of what God claims to stand for. This is the perpetual cry of the child to the parent and the pupil to the teacher: they make demands but deny the means by which these could be satisfied. Adults accuse the child of thinking and behaving wrongly, but they withhold the secret knowledge by which right and wrong may be judged. The child may feel that he is right according to the way he understands things. If the parent or teacher denies the validity of his judgement, then it is because they have not given him the knowledge by which he could have made a better assessment.

Job assumes that he has been right all along. His protestations rise to a pinnacle:

> I will maintain the rightness of my cause, I will never give up;
> so long as I live, I will not change.   (27: 6)

And yet it is here that Job goes on to develop the picture of the fate of the wicked man, which is so closely linked with his own personal experience.

The next chapter (28), which in the New English Version is entitled "God's unfathomable wisdom", can be seen as a swing in Job's thinking towards the idea of a God totally unrelated to any concept which man may produce. Job begins with a metaphor about precious metals which are buried deep in the earth. The imagery of treasures which are buried, and hidden from human sight, can be seen as a metaphor concerning the richness of the being of God which is always hidden from man's understanding.

> There are mines for silver
> and places where men refine gold;
> . . .
> While corn is springing from the earth above,
> what lies beneath is raked over like a fire,
> and out of its rocks comes lapis lazuli,
> dusted with flecks of gold.   (28: 2–6)

The deep veins of buried treasures lie below and are quite unrelated to the human activities which take place on the surface of the earth. It is necessary to go deep under the earth to find gold, silver, and other precious metals, just as it is necessary to go below the surface of conscious thoughts in order to discover the most profound truths.

Wisdom is buried even deeper than the mines in which we find material wealth:

> But where can wisdom be found?
> And where is the source of understanding?
> No man knows the way to it;

> it is not found in the land of living men.
> The depths of ocean say, "It is not in us",
> and the sea says, "It is not with me."
>   (26: 12–14)

There are many legends, myths, and archetypal accounts of a quest which may be symbolized by some hidden material treasure but which represents wisdom in its ultimate purity. It is not obtainable by worldly wealth, and value cannot be put to it:

> Red gold cannot buy it,
> nor can its price be weighed out in silver;
> it cannot be set in the scales against gold of Ophir,
> . . .
> it cannot be set in the scales against pure gold.
>   (26: 15–19)

Job comes to the conclusion that no creature on earth—animal or man—has the key to wisdom and understanding. Only God "understands the way to it,/he alone knows its source" (26: 23). Job, being Job, realizes that his discovery that the acknowledgement that he has not the key to wisdom is, in itself, the key to wisdom which had eluded him. He has reached a new level of humility which is going to make him greater than ever before!

> The fear of the Lord is wisdom
> and to turn from evil is understanding.
>   (26: 28)

Wisdom is not claiming that one has all the wisdom, as the comforters and Job himself had so smugly been doing. There is a balance and proportion in nature, but it is not the moral balance where rewards and punishments can be measured like gold and silver. It is, instead, a kind of self-limiting but all-pervading force throughout nature which only God can fathom:

> When he made a counterpoise for the wind
> and measured out the waters in proportion,
> when he laid down a limit for the rain
> and a path for the thunderstorm,
> even then he saw wisdom and took stock of it,
> he considered it and fathomed its very depths.
>   (28: 25–27)

So far, Job had been considering a balance in nature in terms of material rewards for his own actions. His was a man-centred ideology and was related to the possessions and the fate of man. He is now becoming aware of a different kind of balance. The forces of nature have a strange sort of equilibrium, far beyond man's comprehension, which is represented partly in regularly repeating cycles—like the revolution of the planets which are predictable—and partly by the elemental forces of tempest, earthquakes, and exploding stars which appear to be beyond limit—and yet the universe continues to exist. On earth, the tides advance and recede; there are storms and they subside; rains come to an end. The powers of nature which seem to have the strength to end our world are seen to go only so far and then no farther. There seems to be a self-limiting aspect in this balance of extreme power, yet there is no knowledge of the nature of this force, nor of the agent which controls it. The forces are enormous, but they have their limits. They are beyond man's comprehension; we can only allude to them. Wisdom resides in an awareness of the existence of forces which can never be completely understood. This point relates to man's position in the universe, and also to man's idea of his own mind and of the forces within it.[8] Job now realizes that there are some things even within man himself that can remain beyond human understanding.

Job's final survey of his case is, chapter by chapter, the chronological sequence of his life. He contemplates his progress from childhood and youth to the prosperity of his early adult life (chapter 29); the misery of his present state (chapter 30); and, finally, he recapitulates his continued protestation of innocence (chapter 31).

Job begins chapter 29 with a description of his childhood:

> If I could only go back to the old days,
> to the time when God was watching over me,
> when his lamp shone above my head,
> and by its light I walked through the darkness!
> (29: 2-3)

Job is describing feelings which are similar to those afforded by a protecting and caring mother. His nostalgia for the security of his early adult

---

[8] See our discussion of Elihu (32: 18), p. 115.

home shows a new recognition that his previous life had good aspects which he had been ignoring:

> If I could be as in the days of my prime,
> when God protected my home,
> while the Almighty was still there at my side,
> and my servants stood round me,
> while my path flowed with milk,
> and the rocks streamed oil!   (29: 4–6)

This feeling of complete protection, which is the privilege enjoyed by the rich man in adult life, is an experience of the population as a whole in a brief period of childhood.

The remaining verses of this chapter (29: 7–22) show that he no longer needs to wish the whole of his life away. At the height of his depression, Job had cursed the day he was born, and had wished never to have existed. We have shown how this is related to feelings of loss of that which was good. Now he is able to return in thought to the good times of his nurturing, and to realise that much of what he then possessed had in fact been good. He recounts all the good acts which he had performed, and recalls that he had reckoned on the fullness of his life being everlasting.

> I thought, "I shall die with my powers unimpaired
> and my days uncounted as the grains of sand,
> with my roots spreading out to the water
> and the dew lying on my branches,
> with the bow always new in my grasp
> and the arrow ever ready to my hand."
>   (29: 18–20)

But the very fact that Job had counted on his good acts being rewarded in this manner made it almost inevitable that they would not be. If, in a morally determined world, a good deed were carried out in order to get a reward in heaven, the self-seeking nature of the intention could be weighed against the value of the goodness in the action. A more sophisticated idea of moral justice takes into consideration the intention of an act. An altruistic act would then account for more than an act which is carried out for the sake of reward. From his own experience, Job should have been able to recognize that good acts carried out in the intention of later reward do not amount to much in the end. His own present suffering is a

living example of the uncertainty of the reward for good deeds. But he is
still far from relinquishing his claims.

In chapter 30, Job recognizes that the good did not continue and describes his present feeling of persecution:

> But now I am laughed to scorn
> by men of a younger generation,
>   (30: 1)

Although he is now better able to make a more coherent and reasoned
résumé of his past, the old symptoms return. First the paranoia:

> Now I have become the target of their taunts,
> my name is a byword among them.
> They loathe me, they shrink from me,
> they dare to spit in my face.   (30: 9–10)

Secondly, the psychoneurotic anxieties:

> Terror upon terror overwhelms me,
> 't sweeps away my resolution like the wind,
> and my hope of victory vanishes like a cloud.
> So now my soul is in turmoil within me,
> and misery has me daily in its grip.
>   (30: 15–16)

Thirdly, the psychosomatic symptoms reappear:

> By night pain pierces my very bones,
> and there is ceaseless throbbing in my veins;
> my garments are all bespattered with my phlegm,
> which chokes me like the collar of a shirt.
> . . .
> My bowels are in ferment and know no peace;
> . . .
> My blackened skin peels off,
> and my body is scorched by the heat.
>   (30: 17–18, 27, 30)

It was really too much to hope that all the understanding which Job
had achieved could be either consistent or permanent. Job has not as yet
achieved his cure. But there is a positive factor: even a temporary alleviation of symptoms and a temporary access to wisdom provide a foundation
for future progress and final cure, even if the symptoms should transi-
torily return. If something better has once been experienced, the hope

remains, throughout subsequent regressions, that improvement can be experienced again. Job had reached a greater understanding (chapter 28), and an alleviation of symptoms, and recognition of the good of former days (chapter 29), only to return to the persecutory feelings and physical symptoms (chapter 30). Nevertheless, the possibility has now been established that a cure can in the end be attained.

Chapter 31 is the last and one of the longest of Job's speeches. It is followed only by the intrusion of Elihu and the apparition of God. The chapter is a monumental protest by Job of his innocence, accomplished, in the best manner of perfectionism, by listing all the moral laws which he could have disobeyed, but did not. The obsessional person, who does nothing but good, knows all the wrongs that he could have been doing but for his perfection!

He begins by asking yet again for some kind of equation by which God determines how he is to mete out justice:

> What is the lot prescribed by God above,
> the reward from the Almighty on high?
>
> (31: 2)

He reverts to the traditional moral balance sheet with an all-seeing God as the accountant who tots up every sin against the appropriate punishment:

> Is not ruin prescribed for the miscreant
> and calamity for the wrongdoer?
> Yet does not God himself see my ways
> and count my every step?   (31: 3–4)

Job had earlier reached a new idea of a God less personal than that purported by the comforters. This present reversal in Job's idea of God comes from Job's continued need to show that his suffering is unjustified because his actions had always been right. Job is placing himself back into the double bind from which he cannot yet escape, given the logic of moral accountancy. Although he claims that he should not be suffering, for the reason that he has not sinned, the fact is that he *is* suffering. Therefore, within the terms of his present reasoning, either he must have sinned or God is being deliberately unjust. Job's dilemma continues: he has not as yet successfully extricated himself from the self-defeating reasoning which has guided his continuous protestation of innocence.

He goes on to list all the sins of which he has not been guilty, and this amounts to a recital of the commandments of the early scriptures. Job can check off the prohibitions and asserts that he has transgressed none of them. Never has he had "dealings with falsehood" (31: 5), never committed adultery either in his heart (31: 1), or in fact (31: 9), never ignored the plight of his slaves (30: 13), never withheld support from the needy (31: 17–20), never borne false witness against an innocent (31: 21), never put faith in idols (31: 24–27), never ignored the Mosaic laws concerning the use of the land (31: 38). Not only had he been scrupulous about the letter of the law, but he had also steadfastly maintained the spirit of the law: he has never taken pleasure in the ruin of another man (such as the comforters may secretly have felt at the sight of his own suffering); he has never closed the door of his house to strangers; he has never concealed his misdeeds (if indeed any could be found). Job paints a picture of himself as a good, generous, kindly, totally ethical man, a paragon of virtue. In this day and age he would have been thought too good to be true. The very recounting of his goodness would have provoked his listener to ask what it was that he was covering up. On a psychological level, it might have been described in such jargon terms as "exaggerated superego activity indicating the existence of an excess of guilt feelings".

Even at a conscious level Job himself admits that what had kept him from committing any of these sins was not any particular innate sense of justice, but the fear of God:

> But the terror of God was heavy upon me,
> and for fear of his majesty I could do none of these things.
> (31: 23)

Job is implying that he upheld the laws only because he was afraid that God would punish him if he transgressed them. This would indicate that his goodness was imposed from outside, and not from an inner conviction of the rightness of good acts. Like the child who behaves well only because he fears the reprisals of a stern parent, Job is revealing that his former goodness was not such an integral part of his personality as he had claimed. It was a mode of behaviour deliberately carried out in order to avoid the wrath of God.

Nonetheless, the self-centred quality of Job's attitude enables him to bring God down to the level of an equal contestant. He bargains with God regarding the appropriate punishment that he would accept if God should prove his case. He states that if God could bring proof that Job had transgressed any of the prohibitions which he has so painstakingly listed, then it would be permitted to God to punish him in the following prescribed manner:

> may another eat what I sow,
> and may my crops be pulled up by the roots!
> . . .
> may my wife be another man's slave,
> and may other men enjoy her.
> . . .
> then may my shoulder-blade be torn from my shoulder,
> my arm be wrenched out of its socket!
> . . .
> may thistles spring up instead of wheat,
> and weeds instead of barley!   (31: 8, 10, 22, 40)

Two important factors arise from the listing of these oaths. First, Job relates the kind of punishment that he would be willing to undergo to the type of sin committed. For example, if he had committed adultery, then he would consider it justifiable for God to punish him by submitting his wife to another man's embrace;[9] similarly, if he had not guided his hand to give generously to the needy, then he would consider a just punishment to be the loss of his right hand. In this he is making an abstraction from the traditional idea of proportionate justice. He is ready to sacrifice a hand, not only for what the hand did wrong, but also for what it neglected to do right. Secondly, he is still trying to control God by adjudicating the type of punishment which each transgression would call for. God becomes yet again a force controllable by the laws which he had committed to man.

Job still clings to his original desire to meet God in a court of law in order to defend the righteousness of his cause. Indeed, the very last verse of his final speech ends with a repetition of this wish:

> I would plead the whole record of my life
> and present that in court as my defence.
>   (31: 37)

---

[9] The use of his wife's virtue as a stake in Job's own bargain with God is an instance of his self-centred and male-centred universe. This attitude will change (see Chapter 7).

But in order to hold on to his idea of the integrity of his perfect life, he condemns himself to a battle with God which in reality he has already lost. On the positive side, the fact that he chose to fight the battle is one factor which has kept him from being totally engulfed in his misery. But to reach a state of mind in which he will finally emerge from the suffering is another matter still. However, it is true to say that Job is now looking to a future.

We have seen that Job needs to go beyond that which is traditionally accepted as religious wisdom. The very punishments which he has challenged God to heap on him are made against present or future resources. This must mean that somehow he has found the capital by which to speculate against God once again. It might come as a surprise that Job could wager any possessions if, indeed, he had lost everything which he had previously owned. This, however, is the universal experience of all who succeed in rising from the depths of depression. In the course of psychiatric treatment, a patient who previously had felt to have lost bodily health, possessions, and rectitude begins to find resources of which he had been unaware during the severity of the illness. He makes a discovery of hidden assets, and a redistribution occurs in the qualities of goodness and badness within the personality. The individual can then reassess his past, present, and the possible future resources. Job has now made a reassessment of his past and his present, has been able to take into account the existence of future resources, but he is still firm in his determination to venture all that he has in a contest which is no longer relevant.

Job is certainly correct at one level: God himself had never challenged Job's actions nor made any specific indictment against him: "Let the Almighty state his case against me!" (31: 35). If God had done that, Job could have used God's accusations as his defence, knowing that it would have been impossible to find him guilty of committing any actual sins.

> If my accuser had written out his indictment,
> I would not keep silence and remain indoors.
> No! I would flaunt it on my shoulder
> and wear it like a crown on my head;
> I would plead the whole record of my life
> and present that in court as my defence.
>
> (31: 35–37)

Job would not have hidden himself from an accuser. He would have boldly taken the script of his indictment which he could disprove, as the testimony to his character. Having been found not guilty in open court after a searching inquiry, his character would be seen more clearly to be faultless than that of a man whose deeds had never come under scrutiny.[10] Job's life is his defence, it is his testimonial, and, to this extent, Job is justified in continuing his battle. However, in any contest with God, a mere mortal will lose. In so far as Job is turning the contest into a game of skill,[11] he is putting his cards on the wrong table. God will not answer Job on Job's own terms.

And so the speeches of Job come to an end. His account of his illness and his defence of his innocence are concluded. In the remaining eleven chapters of the narrative, Job is to speak no more than six verses. Just as he reached a deadlock with the comforters, so has he reached a deadlock in his attempt to argue with God. He has set his case proudly; but God does not choose to answer Job's points.[12]

This does not mean that there is no further development in the course of Job's illness and its cure. On the contrary, three episodes in the process of the cure are now to occur. These are the interlude of the speeches of Elihu (a character newly introduced in the Job drama), the intervention of God, and the final reinstatement of Job as described in the Epilogue.

[10] In the field of mental illness not many years ago, when treatment was mostly carried out compulsorily under certification, there were those who looked upon their discharge papers as a certificate of sanity. Occasionally, such a discharged patient would brandish his papers in the course of an argument with someone who had never been through the process of certification, and ask, "Where is *your* certificate?"

[11] See Chapter 7.

[12] This calls to mind Christ's cry during his final agony, "Lord, why hast thou forsaken me." There was no answer. In Alfred de Vig..y's poem, *Le Mont des Oliviers* (1843), Christ bereft of support from his sleeping apostles (as Job is now bereft of the support of his so-called comforters), questions God on the destiny of mankind and on the meaning of his own personal agony. He receives no reply. De Vigny draws a different conclusion about the *silence eternél de la Divinité* from that implied in the Job story. It is interesting to see that the questions of human suffering and the lack of any final support from the outside is a recurring human agony.

CHAPTER 7

The Price of His Release

ELIHU makes his first appearance in chapter 32, following on the final speeches of Job from chapters 26 to 31. Addressing first Job singly, and next Job and the comforters collectively as a group, Elihu holds his audience through the duration of a speech which runs uninterruptedly for six chapters. He is an intruder, an outsider, who, like Camus' Mersault in *L'Etranger*, comes with a message because he is able to see the human dilemma (of which Job is the example) in a different light. The message which he brings contains the rationale which enables Job to be released from his illness.

At the beginning of chapter 32, any group feeling which might have existed between Job and the comforters had been dissipated because they had failed to reach any common ground in their dispute. What transpired between them was scarcely dialogue; it was little more than collective monologue. The arguments were exhausted because the comforters had remained steadfast in their aim to compel Job to confess himself in the wrong, while Job remained steadfast in his aim to prove himself in the right. For all intents and purposes they had failed to communicate.

> So these three men gave up answering Job, for he continued to think himself righteous. (32: 1)

It is at this point that the first mention of Elihu is made:

> Then Elihu, son of Barakel the Buzite, of the family of Ram, grew angry; angry because Job had made himself out more righteous than God, and angry with the three friends because they had found no answer to Job and had let God appear

wrong. Now Elihu had hung back while they were talking with Job because they were older than he; but, when he saw that the three had no answer, he could no longer contain his anger. So Elihu son of Barakel the Buzite began to speak: (32: 2–6)

The Hebrew name "Elihu" means "he is my God", so that Elihu could be thought of as representing the voice of God speaking to Job. In so far as Job has no ready answer to the young intruder, we may understand that he is receptive to what Elihu is saying. His very youthful presence and the new message which he brings are crucial to Job's further development. Our contention is that Job gains something positive from Elihu, both from his words and from the fact that the youthfulness of Elihu transfuses Job with the strength to admit his relative weakness. Job does not even try to out-argue Elihu or beat him into submission. Job is master of his peers, but has to give way eventually to the younger generation.

The two attributes which are applied to Elihu when he is introduced into the narrative are that he is young, and that he is angry. As with the youth of any culture, in any age, he believes that he has a new message and better answers to problems than have his elders. Elihu is the young revolutionary, full of enthusiasm for what he feels to be true, and impatient with his elders for not understanding what is so readily comprehensible to him:

> I am young in years,
> and you are old;
> that is why I held back and shrank
> from displaying my knowledge in front of you.
> . . .
> it is not only the old who are wise
> or the aged who understand what is right.
> . . .
> Look, I have been waiting upon your words,
> listening for the conclusions of your thoughts,
> . . .
> but not one of you refutes Job or answers his arguments.
>
> (32: 6–12)

He is so full of enthusiasm for his new message that he can no longer contain himself. His body is ready to burst under the pressure of his thoughts:

> I will express my opinion;
> for I am bursting with words,

a bellyful of wind gripes me.
My stomach is distended as if with wine,
bulging like a blacksmith's bellows;
I must speak to find relief,
I must open my mouth and answer;

(32: 17–20)

In venturing to speak in contradiction to the views of his elders, Elihu had to overcome the respect for tradition. By the very same action, he was challenging the basis on which the arguments of the comforters had rested. By challenging the elders as persons, he challenged the foundation of their belief that wisdom comes with age and that it is handed down by elders to elders.

If these men are confounded and no longer answer,
if words fail them,
am I to wait because they do not speak,
because they stand there and no longer answer?

(32: 15–16)

Elihu is about to overthrow the old order of polite deference of the young towards the elderly. He is out to find the truth, and will flatter neither man nor God in his searching:

I will show no favour to anyone,
I will flatter no one, God or man;

(32: 21)

In his commitment to answer Job with truth, he will rely upon the confidence which he gains from his own intuition and from the immediacy of his inspiration, and not upon the wisdom derived from the habits of religious tradition:

Look, I am ready to answer;
the words are on the tip of my tongue.
My heart assures me that I speak with knowledge,
and that my lips speak with sincerity.
For the spirit of God made me,
and the breath of the Almighty gave me life.

(33: 2–4)

Elihu's invocation of truth, which comes from the inner quest of man's spirit, picks up a theme which had begun earlier in the narrative. Eliphaz had told of visions which had come to him in the night; Job himself had claimed the right to free association; but in the first instance Eliphaz was unable to carry his vision further than a reaffirmation of traditional religious knowledge, and in Job's case he had, at that point, remained bogged down in his claim to perfection. In contrast we may look upon the message of Elihu as containing the seeds of a new outlook. He begins with new premises:

> In God's sight I am just what you are;
> I too am only a handful of clay.
>
> (33: 6)

Since all men are mortal, the conclusion is that they can avoid the dispute about who is better and who is worse, who is guilty and who is free of guilt. This affirmation is integral to Elihu's later formulation: the abandonment of moral determinacy is required in order to come to terms with human suffering. In one swoop Elihu puts all the participants in the group on to the same plane by putting them all below God. The result of recognizing the equality of standing is an opportunity to dispel one of the grounds for paranoia:

> Fear of me need not abash you,
> nor any pressure from me overawe you.
>
> (35: 7)

Elihu presents no threat. He makes no claim to any special authority, either from the wisdom and experience which derive from age (in contrast with the comforters), nor does he claim the righteousness of perfect behaviour (in contrast with Job). His words can stand on their own. They are not tied to his person. The logic and wisdom of his words will stand or fall on the meaning that they contain.

Several times Elihu invites Job to answer him, but surprisingly Job never takes up the challenge or the opportunity. He is in fact reduced to silence. This is now the third occasion that Job's response to a situation is to maintain a silence. Elihu taunts him:

> Answer me if you can,
> marshal your arguments and confront me.
>
> (33: 5)

11

My bones are pierced in me in the
night season & my sinews
take no rest

My skin is black upon me
& my bones are burned
with heat

The triumphing of the wicked
is short, the joy of the hypocrite is
but for a moment

Satan himself is transformed into an Angel of Light & his Ministers into Ministers of Righteousness

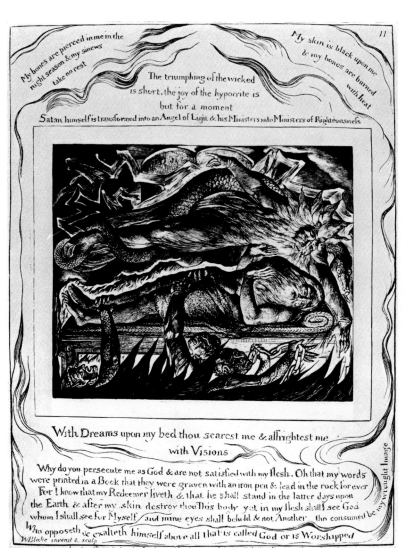

With Dreams upon my bed thou scarest me & affrightest me
with Visions

Why do you persecute me as God & are not satisfied with my flesh. Oh that my words
were printed in a Book that they were graven with an iron pen & lead in the rock for ever
For I know that my Redeemer liveth & that he shall stand in the latter days upon
the Earth & after my skin destroy thou This body yet in my flesh shall I see God
whom I shall see for Myself and mine eyes shall behold & not Another tho consumed be my wrought Image

Who opposeth & exalteth himself above all that is called God or is Worshipped

W Blake invent & sculp

London Published as the Act directs March 8. 1825 by Will Blake N 3 Fountain Court Strand

Proof

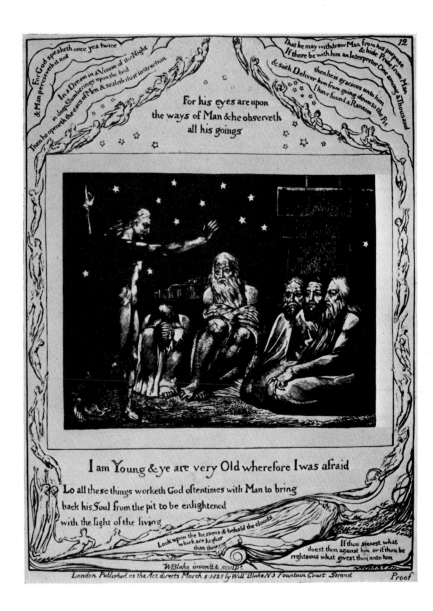

12

For God speaketh once yea twice & Man perceiveth it not

In a Dream in a Vision of the Night in deep Slumberings upon the bed

Then he openeth the ears of Men & sealeth their instruction

That he may withdraw Man from his purpose & hide Pride from Man

If there be with him an Interpreter One among a Thousand

then he is gracious unto him & saith Deliver him from going down to the Pit I have found a Ransom

For his eyes are upon
the ways of Man & he observeth
all his goings

I am Young & ye are very Old wherefore I was afraid

Lo all these things worketh God oftentimes with Man to bring
back his Soul from the pit to be enlightened
with the light of the living

Look upon the heavens & behold the clouds which are higher than thou

If thou sinnest what doest thou against him, or if thou be righteous what givest thou unto him

WBlake invenit & sculpt

London, Published as the Act directs March 8: 1825 by Will: Blake N 3 Fountain Court Strand

Proof

And later,

> If you have any arguments, answer me;
> speak, and I would gladly find you proved right;
> (33: 32)

But Job has nothing to say in reply.

We have already mentioned the importance of the three silences which Job keeps in so far as they are indicative of stages in the illness and the therapeutic process.[1] The first occurred at the beginning of the narrative, when, immediately after the series of calamities and his affliction with sore boils, Job remained silent for seven days and nights. This silence was a measure of the enormity of the losses to which he had been subjected. This silence marked the onset of his breakdown. The second silence occurred at the end of the third cycle of speeches, when, after the comforters had been rendered impotent, Job, in reviewing his case, reached the dilemma from which there seemed to be no escape. This was the silence of exhaustion and emphasized the impasse at which Job and the comforters had arrived. For the comforters, it was an acknowledgement of their unanticipated failure to maintain a moral superiority over someone who had been stripped of the sources of esteem. For Job, the silence was the realization that he could not relinquish his demand on God to meet him in open court on equal terms, and yet he was becoming aware of the futility of his claim. The present (and third) silence which Job will keep during the entire duration of Elihu's speech is an indication that, for the first time, Job is paying attention to what someone else is saying. Nowhere does Job make any direct reply to Elihu, but twice does he make acknowledgement to God. Job is listening from a new centre in himself. It is our contention that it is the message of Elihu which Job will internalize, incorporating it in the resources which he will bring to his final cure.

The first silence and the third silence have something in common. In the first, Job allowed the illness to come through to him and take shape. During the third silence, Job settles his inner conflicts and his further development. The first acknowledged the illness; the third acknowledged

---

[1] This is also true of Job's body positions: the early prostration; the sitting posture which he still maintains; and finally the upright, standing position which God will exhort him to take.

the way to recovery. In this sense, the third silence is creative and healthy. The entrance of Elihu indicates the beginning of a new stage in the course of Job's recovery from his illness.

Considering that Job had such ready answers to all the tirades of his comforters, there must have been something relevant to Job in what Elihu said for him to have remained silent for so long. We have already noticed that Elihu had brought Job, the comforters, and himself all onto an equal level. In so doing, he introduced the concept that God is of a different dimension from man. Elihu now points out that Job had been arguing as if God were someone to be put at fault for making him suffer:

> "I am innocent," you said, "and free from offence,
> blameless and without guilt.
> Yet God finds occasions to put me in the wrong
> and counts me his enemy;
> he puts my feet in the stocks
> and keeps a close watch on all I do".   (33: 9–11)

Job had been searching for a rationale for his suffering within the principles of moral determinacy, but Elihu points out that the causation of human suffering cannot be argued out with God in human terms:

> Well, this is my answer: You are wrong.
> God is greater than man;
> why then plead your case with him?
> for no one can answer his arguments.
> (33: 12–13)

God is not answerable to man in the way that man is answerable to himself for his idea of God. The ways of God are beyond human logic. It is a difference of kind, and not of degree. Job had granted that God was more powerful, along with many other attributes (9: 6–24). All the attributes were human.[2]

Elihu's message to Job is that where his error lay was in looking for the justification of his suffering within the terms of human understanding, wherein Job thought wisdom was to be discovered. Job, being morally correct, had found no logical basis for his suffering. Job had called God to

---

[2] Maimonides (*op. cit.*, pp. 59–64), in discussing the existence of God, points out that certain human qualities are figuratively ascribed to God, but the nature of God in its essence is defined by the absence of any positive attributes. We can say what God is not, but can never define God by what he is.

account within the meaning of the moral laws. The "wisdom" of this logic made Job a man of pride before God. Elihu's contention is that the wisdom which understands the existence of human suffering transgresses the bound of human logic, and that God cannot be worn down by the argument of persistent statement and counter-statement.

> Indeed, once God has spoken
> he does not speak a second time to confirm it.
> (33: 14)

We must not look for the meaning of suffering in the conscious and conscientious ruminations over moral debits and credits, but in the promptings of our unconscious centre:

> In dreams, in visions of the night,
> when deepest sleep falls upon men,
> while they sleep on their beds, God makes them listen,
> and his correction strikes them with terror.
> (33: 15–16)

What kind of event can elicit this understanding? What type of experience can sweep aside the defences of pride? Not man's reliance on his ability to argue logically with God, and win, which in fact separates man from wisdom. Elihu offers an hypothesis of his own:

> To turn a man from reckless conduct,
> to check the pride of mortal man,
> at the edge of the pit he holds him back alive
> and stops him from crossing the river of death.
> Or again, man learns his lesson from a bed of pain,
> tormented by a ceaseless ague in his bones;
> he turns from his food with loathing
> and has no relish for the choicest meats;
> his flesh hangs loose upon him,
> his bones are loosened and out of joint,
> his soul draws near to the pit,
> his life to the ministers of death.   (33: 17–22)

It is the suffering brought on by nearness to the ultimacy of death. It is the intensity of the experience which Job has barely survived. The pride of mortal man is a defence against, or a barrier to, true wisdom and understanding. One has to go to the extremities of life or the borderland of death or insanity to gain the wisdom which repudiates the false logic of causality in the moral sphere. The understanding gained through suffering can bring about release from the burden of attributing responsibility for suffering.

> Yet if an angel, one of thousands, stands by him,
> a mediator between him and God,
> to expound what he has done right
> and to secure mortal man his due;
> if he speaks in the man's favour and says, "Reprieve him,
> let him not go down to the pit, I have the price of his release";
>
> (33: 23–24)

This is a crucial passage which relates to Job's imminent recovery from his illness. Elihu is referring to the vehicle which provides the means for the sufferer to progress from the state of preoccupation with suffering to a level which transcends suffering. According to Elihu, this progress is only possible through the agency of a mediator—the angel who comes unbidden, fortuitously, and as an act of grace. It is of a dimension outside the boundaries of human rationality. We can think here of the role of the "guardian angel" who is the protector of an individual against the chance events which fate may bring into his life. The angel is a mediator between man and God, between man and his fate, and between man and his inner nature. It is this role of mediator, or interpreter,[3] which is relevant here.

Man needs a mediator between that part of himself which suffers, be it physically or psychologically (or both), and that part of himself (which some may call God) which gives him the ability to be released from that suffering. The mediator is the activator of existing potentials.

In another age such a source of change might be seen as the *confidant*, as in drama, who provides a sounding board against which the protagonist can test his thoughts; or figuratively as a midwife who helps to deliver a new life; or the friend who is willing to stand by even if there is no call upon him to intervene. In our present day the psychotherapist may be the one who is seen both as the interpreter and as the helper who creates an atmosphere of faith in the task of healing. He also provides for reparation for that which has been lost, so that the sufferer can feel secure enough to undertake the task of changing and beginning life anew. On another

---

[3] It is interesting to note that in the Authorized Version Elihu's word is rendered as "interpreter", and this bears out the meaning which we are giving to this passage.

level the mediator could be looked upon as the healthy and creative part of the individual which has always been there, dormant though it might be during the period of suffering, which provides the resources (the capital) which the individual may use as energy to invest in the task of change.

Elihu is speaking within the medium of religious understanding of the Old Testament. We are translating this medium into language whose currency may be better understood in the present day. Yet the similarities cannot be overlooked. The idea of the angel, or mediator, who establishes a bridge of understanding between man and God is not so very different from the idealized therapist who represents the symbol of integration between the split parts of the individual's personality, or that part of the individual himself which acts as a source of his own nurturing and growth. Furthermore, the attributes which Elihu gives to the angel are those of CONFIDENCE IN THE EXISTENCE OF GOODNESS IN THE SUF-FERER, THE ABILITY TO IDENTIFY WHAT THE GOODNESS IS, THE WIL-LINGNESS TO BEAR WITNESS IN THE SUFFERER'S FAVOUR, AND THE KNOWLEDGE THAT THE RESOURCES OF CURE ARE PRESENT. The un-deviating faith in the possibility of deliverance cannot be over-emphasized. No less important is the physical presence of the helping agent who is willing to make an effort along with the individual. The comforters had come to Job prepared to go through the process of grief with him. But when Job did not accept their solutions to the question of his suffering, they withdrew their support. It is not Elihu as such, who is offering that support to Job at the present time since he too disagrees with Job's argu-ments. What he *is* offering is the belief in the possibility of finding the right kind of help. It is Elihu's faith that there is a source of help available, and his communication is an explanation of the way in which this help can bridge the gap between the sufferer and his recovery. Job remains silent; he must be accepting Elihu's contribution to his cure.

The mediator, speaking in the sufferer's favour, indicates that the price of release from his suffering is available. This phrase, "the price of his release", is critical to the understanding not only of the importance of Elihu's message but also to the way in which Job will recover from his illness. The price of release in Hebrew is translated from the root word *kipper* [כפר], which means atonement. In the Jewish festival of Yom Kippur, [יום כפור], or the Day of Atonement, sins are collectively confessed and repented, and the festival can be seen as the ritualized or symbolic recognition of the existence of the bad parts of the person. *Kipper* literally means to wipe out, and is related to the earliest Old Testament blood sacrifices. There followed a successive spiritualization of atonement until, at the time of Ezekiel and Job, the idea of internal atonement for sins meant the possibility of restoration of previous wholeness and regeneration into a new life. For this, the necessity always remained that the individual make a ransom or payment (real or token).

Elihu's message is that the price of release from suffering is the sacrifice which follows on the experience of suffering. Greater wisdom and understanding involves man in a loss of his previous pride in his goodness by recognizing the badness which has always been present. Thus can he find, within the humility which allowed him to recognize his imperfections, a new strength to release him from his suffering.

The idea of atonement, represented by the word *kipper*, was given a concrete form (Leviticus 16: 5–10) in connection with two he-goats respectively being the "sin offering" and the "scapegoat". The sin offering was for the Lord; the scapegoat for Azazel,[4] who was a third force, neither God nor the Devil. Azazel is derived from pre-Biblical folklore and is referred to in the Book of Enoch as part of the story of the fall of the angels. The ransom forming the atonement was paid in part to God and in part (no doubt as an insurance) to more primitive supernatural forces holding sway over sexual emotions and rebellious strivings.[5]

[4] Our references to Azazel (Leviticus, Authorized Version, 16) are drawn from the *Jewish Encyclopedia*, Vol. 11 (New York: Funk & Wagnall's, 1902), pp. 365–367. The word "Azazel" is taken directly from the Hebrew text, but in the Authorized Version it would appear that the translators were concerned more with giving an account of the ceremony than a literal translation, and rendered the Hebrew word as scapegoat. The Revised Version gives "Azazel"; the New English Version speaks of "the goat for the Precipice", thus referring to its fate, but gives "Azazel" as a footnote.

[5] This again calls to mind the depiction of Christ as the "lamb of God", a symbol of perfection offered to God to expiate the sins of mankind. Only a perfect and flawless creature was considered appropriate as a sacrifice to God, and this has allusions to Job's own perfection and his subsequent suffering. Job could be considered as the perfect victim for sacrifice to God, but the deeper level which we are attempting to uncover here is that there are various dimensions to being perfect, and that each has its own consequences.

For early Scriptural references to the flawlessness of the sacrificial lamb, see Exodus 12: 5 and Leviticus 5: 15. The New English Version translates the root word *tam* as "without blemish". In our earlier discussion, this same word was

There is a similarity between the idea of atonement of sins and the suffering undergone in a physical or mental illness. It is a popular idea that illness can be enobling to the character, although it is only a minority of people who truly find it so. Many sufferers succumb, and many others are the worse for their experience. And yet a mentally ill person, who is given the chance through therapy to recuperate, may do so by the very understanding and insight which he gains through suffering his illness. The word "suffering" implies not only the experience of pain, but also the idea of "tolerating evil". If an individual can tolerate his own badness, even though it might cost him a good deal of pain in the recognizing that he is not totally good, the suffering acquires a meaning for him and gains an importance in his further maturation.

We do not wish here to glorify illness, which inevitably is a regression. The regression nevertheless can provide a second chance for the individual to go through some of the stages of development which had been missed on the first time round. Survival from physical illness which brings a person near to death can be perceived as a rebirth. When someone who is suffering from depression makes an attempt at suicide and fails, the nearness to death may be sufficient to wipe out the despair which was embodied in the personality that had so nearly destroyed itself.

Such a rebirth is the second chance in which one can begin with a credit of goodness:

> then that man will grow sturdier than he was in youth,
> he will return to the days of his prime,
> If he entreats God to show him favour,
> to let him see his face and shout for joy;
> if he declares before all men, "I have sinned,
> turned right into wrong and thought nothing of it";
> then he saves himself from going down to the pit,
> he lives and sees the light. (33: 25–28)

The former badness is counteracted by the newly found goodness. This theme has been discussed by Melanie Klein:[6]

---

shown to apply to Job (see Chapter 2) in reference to his unblemished moral character, and was compared with his subsequent boils—or blemishes—the outward sign of inner imperfections.

[6] Melanie Klein, *op. cit.*, p. 16.

> The irrevocable fact that none of us is ever entirely free from guilt has very
> valuable aspects because it implies the never fully exhausted wish to make repar-
> ation and to create in whatever way we can.

Job had maintained his righteousness and therefore denied his badness.
His obsessional observances were the means to keep him from seeing the
badness. Elihu points out that the recognition of badness is a precondition
to recovery. If Job can rid himself of the pride which he had had in his
virtue and recognize that, like any other human being, he has a bad side
as well as a good one, then he may reach the very doors of death and yet
survive.

> All these things God may do to a man,
> again and yet again,
> bringing him back from the pit
> to enjoy the full light of life.
>
> (33: 29–30)

Such extremities of experiences may occur repeatedly. The message is one
of hope that a positive outcome is available and that the testing of the
individual again and again is a way for him to gain the wisdom and
understanding of human experiences which lie outside logical interpretation.

Elihu now goes on to address the three comforters as well as Job:

> Mark my words, you wise men;
> you men of long experience, listen to me;
>
> (34: 2)

Elihu exhorts them all to join in a group endeavour to search out the
truth:

> Let us then examine for ourselves what is right;
> Let us together establish the true good.
>
> (34: 4)

He makes them into a group again by using the words "let us . . .". It
would be possible that Job could become more accessible to Elihu's
message by reason of the fact that he will not be singled out to receive it.
As a group phenomenon, this is called "universalization" and helps to reduce
the sense of isolation and shame.[7]

[7] S. Thompson and J. H. Kahn, *The Group Process as a Helping Technique* (Oxford:
Pergamon Press, 1970), p. 63.

Elihu includes Job, as well as himself, in the same group, and thus dispels the experience of separation which had followed on Job's final review of his case. It is also an elaboration of Elihu's message that the path to wisdom involves getting to a common ground, the recognition that all men are the same under God, and that no one man is better than another.

The next task, he asserts, is to examine the problem together. He again reviews the case Job has made for himself (34: 6–9), but answers that Job cannot call upon God to be just if being "just" means that God must act on principles which human beings can decide.

Elihu continues his repudiation of moral determinacy by showing how irrelevant is the whole idea of reward expected for good acts (and punishment for bad ones) in comparison with the understanding that comes from considering the mysteries of the universe:

> Look up at the sky and then consider,
> observe the rain-clouds towering above you.
> How does it touch him if you have sinned?
> However many your misdeeds, what does it mean to him?
> If you do right, what good do you bring him
> or what does he gain from you?
> Your wickedness touches only men, such as you are;
> the right that you do affects none but mortal man.
>
> (35: 5–8)

The last two lines should command special attention. They enclose the key to Job's release from his argument with God. By understanding that human actions can have no effect upon God, man is released from the complexities of a "special relationship" with God. If man, in his idea of God, releases him from accountability within the bounds of moral law, then man also is released from the awful burden of having to call God to account for the evil in the world. Moreover, if man is able to call God to account, then God must be subject to his own creation. If man, the creature, is stronger than God, the creator, then man can no longer look for strength outside his own self.

This theological argument regarding the relationship of human morality to the qualities of the divine being has a practical aspect in the development of the image of the parent in every human infant. The parent at first seems omniscient and omnipotent. It seems to the child that the parent can see into his mind and can carry out actions on an apparently unlimited scale. The child rebels at first in a futile way against the parent's power and intrusions, even while at the same time seeking the benefits and satisfaction of loving care. The fury of the infantile attacks are threatening to the infant's own self. He fears that by attacking the source of badness he will destroy at the same time the source of goodness. Kleinian dynamic psychology postulates that the splitting of goodness and badness occurs in the child's earliest experiences, but that, as he develops, he integrates goodness and badness within himself and can accept those same qualities in the individual upon whom he is dependent. Progress is made when the parent is perceived as no longer omnipotent and omniscient but as still retaining some power to give benefit and impose controls. Part of the child's maturation is the experience that the parent survives his anger and temper tantrums.

Elihu is making it possible for Job to see how, on a theological level, God can survive the anger of man towards him. WHAT ELIHU IS DOING IS ASSURING THE SURVIVAL OF THE IDEA OF A GOD WHO CAN SURVIVE THE RANTINGS OF A JOB. God is no weaker or stronger if Job has sinned or remained righteous: morality is human and adds nothing to God. In so far as Job's illness is related to his sense of moral rectitude, his illness is a purely human affair. The challenge which Job is making against God about the injustices he is suffering is an adult magnification of an infantile phase of psychological development:

> So, when they cry out, he does not answer,
> because they are self-willed and proud,
> All to no purpose! God does not listen,
> the Almighty does not see.

> The worse for you when you say, "He does not see me"!
> Humble yourself in his presence and wait for his word.
> But now, because God does not grow angry and punish
> Job gives vent to windy nonsense
> and makes a parade of empty words.   (35: 12–16)

The good parent does not answer the content of the child's cries, neither need abstract authority answer every complaint (*de minimis non curat lex*). The needs of the developing individual are best served by the protective insurance of the caring body which has confidence in itself.

It is the pride of man which exaggerates the importance even of his misdeeds.

The remainder of Elihu's argument is devoted to the theme of the mysteries of God's works as against a simple system of God's transactions with man:

> All men stand back from him;
> the race of mortals look on from afar.
> Consider; God is so great that we cannot know him;
>   (36: 24–26)

He catalogues some of the natural phenomena which were not understood at the time in scientific terms—thunder, rain, floods, hurricanes, the course of the clouds—to prove that man cannot argue with a God related to such mysteries. It is almost the same language as God's own answer out of the whirlwind. God is outside the style of thought of man. Men therefore pay him reverence:

> But the Almighty we cannot find; his power is beyond our ken,
> and his righteousness not slow to do justice.
> and all who are wise look to him.   (37: 23–24)

Elihu has now finished the argument meant to dissipate the idea of a special relationship binding man to God and God to man. And yet in the line "his righteousness not slow to do justice" he cannot entirely escape from traditional doctrine (neither will Job, nor will subsequent generations of men who attempt to rationalize their religion).

Job now has at hand the means by which he can release himself from the pride involved in maintaining himself in the right while putting God in the wrong. The dissipation of Job's argument constitutes the price of Job's release from his illness. At this point Job has no need to cling to the image of perfection in order to maintain his uprightness before God. Neither does he need to insist upon the magnitude of his deprivations.

Job had not even lost all his children. Reference has already been made to the Septuagint Bible which mentions the children of his concubines The actual verses are:

> When with my mouth I entreated and supplicated my
> wife, and called affectionately to the children of
> my concubines; they renounce me forever. When I
> insist they speak against me.   (19: 17–18)[8]

---

[8] Translation of Charles Thomson (U.S.A: The Falcon's Wing Press, 1954).

Although the point at issue is that Job was complaining of being spurned by his own family, he acknowledges the continued existence of his seed, even if not in the main line of inheritance. By the same token, he is acknowledging the existence of something in his past which the translators of the Authorized Version must have found less than perfect.

In the present context, Elihu finds nothing inappropriate to Job in the imagery of material riches which he employs:

> Beware, if you are tempted to exchange hardship for comfort,
> for unlimited plenty spread before you, and a generous table;
> if you eat your fill of a rich man's fare
> when you are occupied with the business of the law,
> do not be led astray by lavish gifts of wine
> and do not let bribery warp your judgement.
> Will that wealth of yours, however great, avail you,
> or all the resources of your high position?
> Take care not to turn to mischief;
> for that is why you are tried by affliction.   (36: 16–21)

This bears out the fact that throughout the Bible narrative Job has not lost that basic image, which was first presented in the Prologue, of a great man tested. The greatest man in the East has been tested by God and has barely survived. He has survived partly through the very argumentation which he has carried on with God, and yet there was something further to accomplish finally to release him from his suffering. Elihu has provided the "price of his release" while at the same time not reducing the basic image of Job.

In the final chapter of the present book we shall see how Job incorporates the message of Elihu into his own being; this active internationalization will be seen as God's answer to Job from out of the whirlwind.

CHAPTER 8

Tempest of the Mind

THE transition from the speeches of Elihu to God's answer to Job out of the tempest is not prepared for in the Bible text. For all its dramatic introduction, God's argument follows on without perceptible change from that of Elihu. One stops, the other begins: the theme continues.

A superficial interpretation of Job's restoration to health would be that God tells Job what he has been doing wrong, Job acknowledges his error, and is then immediately cured. This is as much a travesty of the Bible story as is the conventional representation of psychiatric treatment on the stage or screen, in which the psychiatrist uncovers an early traumatic experience, which the patient acknowledges, whereupon he is cured.

There is just sufficient truth in the idea that the recapitulation of past events releases emotion, with beneficial effects, to justify the prevalent belief that some particular incident is responsible for the long continued distress of mental disorder. Trilling makes the point that "psychoanalysis is a science which is based upon narration, upon telling. Its principle of explanation consists in getting the story told—somehow, anyhow—in order to discover how it begins. It presumes that the tale that is told will yield counsel."[1]

In psychoanalytical practice, however, it is to the emotional content of the story that is told to which value is attached. The traumatic incidents are projected onto a memory screen which hides still earlier and more primitive aspects of human existence. The conflicts are not extraneous to life, but are part of it; and the treatment is not a removal of

[1] Lionel Trilling, *Sincerity and Authenticity* (London: Oxford University Press, 1972), p. 140.

something alien to the previous normality, but an opportunity for developing some potentialities which hitherto had remained latent. It is in this manner that we connect the speech out of the tempest with the speech of Elihu which preceded it. Job is given the opportunity to pay the price of his release and, in return, he is allowed to regain his former state and further to develop his creativity.

Throughout, Job had been demanding to meet God in a court of law to decide whether his suffering was justified. What is important in the process of the cure is that Job had wanted a confrontation with God on Job's own terms. Part of cure lies in recognizing that things do not go the way one expected. God's first words are:

> Who is this whose ignorant words
> cloud my design in darkness?
> Brace yourself and stand up like a man;
> I will ask questions, and you shall answer.
>   (38: 2-3)

In these verses, three messages are conveyed.

First, God casts aside the arguments which Job had already mustered in his defence within the premises of moral determinacy. God's complete design of the universe is greater than any which could be accounted for in Job's moral system. It is Job's viewpoint which is deficient, and which clouds the larger meanings which are implicit in the vastness of creation. In simple terms, Job is ignorant, and God, like an angry and demanding father, is going to confound him with a cosmic view which will supercede the human ideas of moral determinacy. In this process, Job's comprehension of the mysteries of the universe will be stretched to the limits of his understanding.

Secondly, it is not Job who is going to declare the conditions for confrontation. God will not be made to answer man for the results of his creation. Neither is it within human capacity to envisage a universe of infinite extent. It is God who is coexistent with the un-understandable; it is God who puts man into his subluminary situation. It is for man to react to his own humanness; it is not for man to call God to account for the limitations of concrete, human existence.

Thirdly, God calls upon Job to take the upright position. Throughout the cycle of speeches with the three comforters, and during the intervention of Elihu, Job had remained seated. In the confrontation with God,

Job is to show respect for the Almighty, and respect for himself, by taking responsibility for the "uprightness" of his posture. This is significant in so far as Job led a life which, at the beginning, was described as "upright".

Within our psychodynamic framework, we have been concerned chiefly with the emotional aspects of Job's mental processes. In pre-psychoanalytical psychology this was described as the affective element of mental life. The other two elements were cognition and conation. These latter two elements are sometimes neglected in descriptions of psychotherapy, but they are nonetheless an essential component. Cognition is the intellectual appraisal of the perceptions of the universe. Conation represents man's will to act. In the above verses (38: 2–3) lies an appeal to these two elements. Job is being called upon to question his perceptions of the external world. This is the cognitive aspect. It is his intellectual understanding which is being tested and extended. The command to brace himself and stand up like a man gives the impetus for him to use his new knowledge which gives him the power and the will to action. This is conation. Job's cure will be judged by what he feels (affect), what he thinks (cognition), and, finally, by what he does (conation). The call for muscular activity is an appeal to the physical human being with a backbone which gives man his erect posture. Human action is as important as human thought and human feeling.

Job has not completed his appraisal of his position in the world. The questions which are basic to human existence are turned back to man himself. In Elihu's words: "It is for you to decide, not me:" (34: 33). It will be man who is responsible for matching his perceptions of the external world with his religious and scientific theorizing. God is what is left over after the universe has been explained by the science of any particular age.

God identifies himself (chapters 38–41) with the part of physical and animate nature that is still unknown. This new God, no longer anthropomorphic but still a God of nature, enjoys a power far beyond anything against which man can measure himself. He encloses everything that is still unknown. But the language does not quite capture the concept of the *unknowable* as against the *unknown*. In describing all the expressions of God's power in nature and in the physical universe, a step is being taken towards *making* these things known and towards making them accessible to penetration by man's mind. Describing them reduces somewhat the ultimate unknowable and ineffable nature of a God who is beyond description.

The limits beyond the reach of science are those areas which are the subject of mythology. In the story of the Garden of Eden, the Tower of Babel, and many others, there are certain elements in common. There is an image of a God who is omniscient and omnipotent, who proffers knowledge but prohibits man from reaching out for it. This God's fear is that the searcher for knowledge will inherit his supremacy. Such a God is constructed anthropomorphically, allowing man a blissful state during the period of his ignorance (or innocence), but at the same time giving him precise instructions on how to acquire the knowledge for the possession of which he is to be punished.

The scope of God appears to be reduced by each new step that man takes in the discovery of knowledge of his inner self and of the external universe. New knowledge and new powers in man give him a degree of mastery over his own fate. It takes him into a science where the test of the truth is its power to predict events from previous causes. Man's advance, however, is limited by the extent of the permanently unpredictable, which is far beyond that which is merely unpredicted up to the present date. There are the events which so far remain unpredictable, but which will eventually come under causal laws through the growth of knowledge. Progress up to date has encouraged many scientists to hope that eventually the whole universe, animate and inanimate, will be brought under the inviolate laws which can be clearly laid down. This is a basic error which was able to be maintained by scientists so long as they were dealing with fairly simple formulations in which some observed regularities became dignified by the term "scientific law". As scientific knowledge extends into progressively more complex areas of observation and conceptualization, it has to be recognized that there are some phenomena in which the essential quality is that the operation takes place by chance. It is even possible to construct a machine in which the test of its efficiency is that it produces random results. Such a machine is used to operate for lotteries where chance is the desired aim. Chance is the part of nature which is unknowable and unpredictable, and is to be distinguished from that which is merely unknown or unpredicted. There is much that is unknown which will become known. *The unknown thus becomes reduced.*

The unknowable increases even more rapidly than that which becomes known.
Each increase in knowledge gives man a glimpse of some fragment of the
infinite unknowable, but the content of the unknowable becomes en-
larged.

In so far as human life is influenced in a chance fashion, a further idea
has to be introduced, beyond science and beyond chance, and, as far as
religion is concerned, even beyond theology. This idea is that of *destiny*
which is something that is supernaturally determined. It is destiny which
defeats man's efforts to know or control the forces outside the boundaries
of the currently existing science. It is destiny which relates the Bible stories
of Eden and Babel to the Greek tragedies. A prohibition exists together
with an opportunity to violate it: in the Garden of Eden the tree of knowledge of good and evil (of sexuality) was available, and temptation came
from outside; in the Tower of Babel, the challenge to God was through
technological achievement; in the Oedipus story, the temptation was in
the form of a riddle which is a stimulus to curiosity; in the Prometheus
story, man had the opportunity to steal the power which had hitherto
been the exclusive possession of the gods. These extensions of man's
powers into the unknown are depicted as an arrogant challenge of the
destiny which limits man's permitted performance. The challenge to
destiny is *hubris*, or the pride of man. This pride, which carries man into
the danger of being punished by the gods, is also the spur to change the
terms under which destiny operates. When it is successful it yields its
rewards, but it also carries a penalty of retribution or punishment which is
potentially commensurate with the rewards.

The retribution or punishment is experienced as depression and is
expressed as guilt. Trilling, dealing with psychoanalytical ideas, refers to
conscience and distinguishes it from the *superego*, which is not limited by
logical or rational considerations. The pain inflicted by the tyranny of the
superego is that which Freud calls *guilt*. He points out that Freud distinguishes guilt from *remorse* which is the consciousness of wrongdoing:

> "When one has a sense of guilt after having committed a misdeed, and because
> of it, the feeling should more properly be called *remorse*. It relates only to a
> deed that has been done. . . ."[2]

---

[2] Lionel Trilling (*op. cit.*, p. 152, note 2), quoting Sigmund Freud, "Civilization
and Its Discontents", *Standard Edition*, Vol. XXI (London, 1963), p. 131.

The price of the release from the pain of guilt is some sacrifice of personal esteem (humility), or reparation to some outside being or system. The intermediary—angel or therapist—validates the transition from pride to humility, and facilitates the reparation.

The process is never quite complete. When the transaction is concluded, and reparation has been made, new levels can be achieved, but the new levels are not very much higher than, or very different from, the previous mode of operating. Pride and possessions accumulate once more, and again become the origins of self-esteem. The new Job which will emerge is going to have some very strong resemblances to the old Job!

Present-day progress in science has made it possible to disrupt the integrity of the atom, to alter the chemical composition of living tissue, and to make a physical penetration of outer space. Yet man has still to face some of the issues now raised:

> Where were you when I laid the earth's foundations?
> Tell me, if you know and understand.
> Who settled its dimensions? Surely you should know.
> Who stretched his measuring-line over it?
> On what do its supporting pillars rest?   (38: 4–6)

The manner of God's speech is ironical. God is impressing Job with examples of his power. Jung speculates on the nature of this God who has to have a combat with man and bring in "his whole power machine and parade it before his opponent".[3] Jung's point is that Yahweh is tormented by the fact that a guiltless Job had somehow secretly been lifted up to a knowledge of God superior to that which God himself possessed. Satan comes into this drama as the mischief-making son of God who, in the end, is never brought to account. Nor is Job given the moral satisfaction (in the narrative) of having God's behaviour explained. According to Jung, the passage

> Who is this whose ignorant words
> cloud my design in darkness?
>
> (38: 2)

is inappropriate to Job: "The only dark thing is how Yahweh ever came to make a bet with Satan."[4] In answer to Jung, we would maintain that

[3] C. G. Jung, *op. cit.*, p. 28.
[4] *Ibid.*, pp. 22–24.

clarity comes from regarding the whole drama as taking place within the mind of Job. We grant, with Jung, that there has been a contest between man and his God, but that this is a perpetual contest in which man must ever subordinate himself if his God is to be preserved. Man succeeds to the extent that he alters his God. But guilt, remorse, and reparation supervene.

The rationality behind the speech put into the mouth of God is the continuing and residual mysteries which recede rapidly into the distance as science pursues its knowledge.

> Have the gates of death been revealed to you?
> Have you ever seen the door-keepers of the place of darkness?
> Have you comprehended the vast expanse of the world?
> (38: 17–18)

It is God who puts the limits to the universe, not man:

> Did you proclaim the rules that govern the heavens?
> or determine the laws of nature on earth?   (38: 33)

Job's challenge to God had had the authorization of the concept of moral determinacy and the science of his age. God's oblique reply to this challenge is that mankind, including Job, can never understand the principles which set up the rules guiding natural phenomena. Job had granted that wisdom and understanding lay in fearing God and turning from evil. But for God, this apparent humility of Job does not go far enough:

> Who put wisdom in depths of darkness
> and veiled understanding in secrecy?
> (38: 36)

Only God can see through the secrets and mysteries of the universe, because it was he who created them, and then enveloped them in secrecy.

This God of mystery proclaims the location of his secrets but puts barriers in the way of their discovery. To hide is to invite discovery. It is a seduction to violate the mysteries, and therefore every success must be punished. The God of Genesis, which appears to have been Job's God, has to hold on precariously to his power which is superior to that of man. This concept of God encloses an everlasting truth which is that every discovery of man is accompanied by a potential pain. A new truth is a destruction of an old and familiar truth, and there is a period during which the new truth cannot give security. A new technique may make old techniques obsolete, but the new one may have unforeseen hazards. Nevertheless, the urge to discover, to invent, and to formulate is an essential property of man; and, in this sense, man learns to conquer the God which he inherits from the previous generation. Part, at least, of the pain is the knowledge that the progress is never complete.

Jung has implied that in this narrative Job was in a superior position to God. The superiority can only exist at the moment of some conquest where there is a diminution in what once was God, and which is now human. It is something akin to Freud's saying "Where id was, ego shall be." Neither God nor the unconscious are reducible by the access of some elements to conscious control. When something is subtracted from infinity, infinity still remains. Freud's hope that the unconscious would be reduced by the growth of the conscious was illusory and, in relation to God, man retains his essentially inferior position, even in the aftermath of his greatest conquests. Whereas in the earlier stages of the narrative Job had granted a superior position in a measurable, quantitative sense, we now approach an idea of an unquantifiable God with whom comparison cannot logically be made. Comparisons, nevertheless, still continue to be made and are contained in qualitative differences between man and God, inconsistent though this may be with the insight which had been attained.

This theme continues (chapter 39) when God refers to the wild animals who have offspring without the help which man gives to those which are under his dominion. Man has limited the existence of domestic animals within terms which are human, or which serve human needs. There are animals which are untamable, and beyond the constraints which men may wish to place on them, and the emerging God is of the same category.

If we look upon this speech as a development of the concept of God, we still have the paradox of a God who is detaching himself from the consequences of a covenant with man, but who is still taking the trouble to explain it. Nowhere can man completely remove his God from some element of human shape, but the anthropomorphism is a mere shadow compared with the picture of the God encountered in Genesis. God first created the animal kingdom, next created man in his own image, and then handed to man the dominion over the animals. Man, created in the image of his creator, shared with him some of his authority. And this was the authority which Job assumed when calling upon God to account for the way in which he had imposed suffering on him. Elihu's arguments had been intended to dispel the rationale for this relationship between man and God. The argument is now being elaborated by the reference to the existence of animals outside man's dominion. The novelty of this concept is the recognition that much of the animal world is outside man's kingdom and far exceeds an animal community which could be enclosed in an Ark. The animal world is of infinite dimension, and in this it can be equated with the unconscious forces within man which, like the wildness of nature, are relatable to God. This new God is now beginning to resemble the part of man and the part of nature which is not consciously understood nor is under control.

Implicit in the descriptions (chapters 38–40) is the richness, profusion, and variety of living species and of the forces of nature.[5]

The power of man does not extend to the origin of the strength of animals, even if men uses them for his own purposes:

> Did you give the horse his strength?
> . . .
> Does you skill teach the hawk to use its pinions
> . . .
> Do you instruct the vulture to fly high
> and build its nest aloft?   (39: 19–27)

There are limits to human supremacy in nature:

> Can you pull out the whale with a gaff
> or can you slip a noose round its tongue?
> Can you pass a cord through its nose
> Or put a hook through its jaw?
> Will it plead with you for mercy
> or beg its life with soft words?
> Will it enter into an agreement with you
> to become your slave for life?
> Will you toy with it as with a bird
> or keep it on a string like a song-bird for your maidens?
>   (41: 1–5)

The wild beasts follow laws which man can neither understand nor control. Likewise, God is a law unto himself and cannot be harnessed to the

[5] This picture of the complex variety of species, now being used to remove man from the special position which had been assumed with God, was later used by Darwin to advance the idea that a single act of creation was not credible.

rules by which men live. Job's laws were civilized laws, moral laws, which have to do with the relationship between man and man and between man and a man-like God. But God is now represented in uncivilized, elemental forces and not in the person of man.

God is identified with the wildness of nature, the undomesticatable, untamable, uncontrollable side, which has its resonances with that aspect of man which, being unconscious, is irrational and unpredictable, and which escapes being bound or harnessed by moral laws. Elihu had already established the arbitrary quality of God, as well as his strength which is beyond human control, and this is now being restated.

The postulations which we are advancing involve a reversal of many familiar values. The growth of intellect, of scientific knowledge, and of the use of material resources are valued highly in the scale of human aspirations. Even more highly valued is the idea of human justice, reflecting the justice of a just God. The value of the undiscoverable, the unknowable, has a more elusive appeal, and the ability to relinquish the notion of retributive justice is not fully within human capacity, even though tentative efforts continue to be made to explore these dimensions of uncertainty.

This capacity to reverse traditional values involves some toleration of ambiguity in the use of the words which describe the concepts as they emerge from the mind of man. In these dimensions, the simultaneous use of opposite meanings has to be accomplished.

An instance of this appears in the subtle use of the word "tempest" (38: 1, New English Version; the Authorized Version gives "whirlwind") out of which God makes his proclamations to Job. The same word is used earlier for the forces that bore down upon Job (9: 17). The Authorized Version gives, "For he breaketh me with a tempest." The New English translation does not include the word "tempest" at this point, but the original Hebrew has the same root word in both passages. The tempest which Job experienced as a source of suffering is the same as that which later brought him enlightenment.

All wisdom is achieved with pain. Every interpretation which brings knowledge involves the sacrifice of the satisfaction and security enclosed in existing ways of life. A new interpretation is both an enlargement of ideas and a destruction of previous conceptualizations. The destruction brings the pain; the new insight offers a prospect of hitherto unknown satisfactions. But wisdom does not always bring happiness, and the turmoil of the tempest survives into the period beyond.

Human beings in general grieve for the lost simplicity of olden times and, in their personal lives, for their infancy, their youth, and for the time when maturity was still something to be achieved. This idea is expressed in Ecclesiastes (1: 17–18):

> And I gave my heart to know wisdom, and to know madness and folly: I perceived that this also is vexation of spirit. For in much wisdom is much grief: and he that increaseth knowledge increaseth sorrow.[6]

The simultaneous and successive use of opposites continues within the Job story at this stage. Up until now Job had insisted on his right to be in the right, and, if necessary, to put God in the wrong. But now Job hears the voice of God say,

> Is it for a man who disputes with the Almighty to be stubborn?
> Should he that argues with God answer back?   (40: 2)

Job is tentatively putting himself in the wrong,[7] but the voice in which he hears himself speak is the voice of God. An example of this frequently occurs in the practice of psychiatry. A patient volunteers accusations and recriminations against his own self. If the psychiatrist says to such a patient "Suppose the same criticisms were being made, not by you, but by someone else, in whose voice could you imagine yourself hearing those words?", the answer almost invariably is either "my mother" or "my father". The patient has to put himself in the wrong in order to maintain the rightness of the parent. Nowhere is this process more vehement than in those cases where the parent has imposed unjustified injuries on his own child. The accusations might well have been from the child to the

[6] The New English Version reads:

> So I applied my mind to understand wisdom and knowledge, madness and folly, and I came to see that this too is chasing the wind. For in much wisdom is much vexation, and the more a man knows, the more he has to suffer.

[7] Shakespeare provides a similar example of the self-criticism of a rejected suitor which is necessary to preserve the idealized image of the unattainable lover:

> Such is my love, to thee I so belong
> That for thy right myself will bear all wrong.
> (Sonnet LXXXVIII)

parent, but if voice was given in this direct form, the patient would have to sacrifice the image of a benevolent parent who gives security. So, too, with Job. Only by putting himself in the wrong can he regain the security of shelter in his patriarchal God.

In the former stages of Job's development it would have been possible to put himself in the wrong only by taking on personal guilt, and this would have been difficult for Job with his exaggerated sense of self-righteousness. Indeed, his righteousness had become a challenge to God, and he had all but lost the ensuing combat. Job was able to rescue himself by envisaging a God of a power so immense that the issue of personal guilt had become irrelevant. The progress to this position had been uneven. Several times Job had approached it, only to return to his previous state.

If we were to imagine a living Job, who as a patient had come through a depressive illness to new levels of understanding, we should expect the progress to be uneven. A chronological account would not show a logical sequence of development of thought, nor a coherent pattern in the relief of emotional distress. Even after that which passes for cure, an inner core of archaic patterns of thinking and feeling would remain potentially operative. Change occurs; new levels are attained; but there is a central stream in the continuity of identity.

Job has lost his special relationship with God in his acceptance of the message that God is above such relationships. But in the end he will find some device by which he can preserve a relationship, albeit one that is somewhat different from the original model. It may have seemed sufficient to him to put himself in the wrong in order that he might be able to retain possession of a God who is always in the right.

The very act of cutting away one special relationship and replacing it by another means that the new relationship, like the old one, is a very personal possession. In that sense Job is closer than ever before to the new God, which out of his need he has helped to create. Job has not achieved the position of separating God from the attributes of the physical creation. In identifying God with the wildest aspects of nature, he has liberated him from a close identification with his own self. Job has thus become able to diminish his own personal image and by enlarging God he merges himself with the rest of humanity. At this moment he has become humble. Therefore, can Job answer God:

What reply can I give thee, I who carry no weight?
I put my finger to my lips.
I have spoken once and now will not answer again;
twice have I spoken, and I will do so no more.

(40: 3–5)

These are the first words that Job has spoken since he had ended the recital of his case (chapter 31), still maintaining the certainty of his rightness. The phrase "I who carry no weight" (translated by the Authorized Version as "I am vile") is in complete contrast to the perfection and righteousness which previously he had been claiming. The new-found humility which Job has achieved is part of his cure.

The Hebrew word which has been rendered in the New English Version as "I carry no weight" means, literally, "I am too slight". This word derives from the Hebrew noun for "ignominy" or "dishonour". The idea of shame is closely related to all these words and, seen in the light which Job directs on to himself, it is the opposite of the arrogance which had been attributed to Job in the speeches of Elihu and God.

The idea of shame is used by Erikson in describing the basic task in the stage of acquiring autonomy (or integrity). Erikson states:

> Shame is early expressed in the impulse to bury one's face, or to sink, right then and there, into the ground. But this, I think, is essentially rage turned against the self.[8] (p. 223)

And later:

> He who is ashamed would like to force the world not to look at him, not to notice his exposure. He would like to destroy the eyes of the world. Instead, he must wish for his own invisibility.[9] (p. 223)

Job has "put his fingers to his lips"—he has stopped arguing and is silent. Erikson takes his argument further into the stages of development in childhood where the process of shaming is deliberately introduced by the adult world to maintain its supremacy over each new generation:

> Such shaming exploits an increasing sense of being small, which can develop only as the child stands up and as his awareness permits him to note the relative measures of size and power.[10]

---

[8] Erik H. Erikson, *Childhood and Society* (New York: W.W. Norton & Co., 1950), p. 223.
[9] *Ibid.*   [10] *Ibid.*, p. 223.

Throughout the exhortations from God to Job the import is the smallness of man's power compared with that of God, and the tone carries a note of sarcasm which matches that of Job to his comforters. This message is the second meaning in the command to "stand up like a man". The first time the phrase was used it was an invitation to Job to use his own resources in his recovery. On this occasion it is a reminder to Job of his smallness compared with God. The child who stands up to his full height not only increases his stature but also demonstrates the smallness of it on the adult scale. To extend himself gives pride and pleasure, but the sacrifice of the illusion of adult size gives pain—and the potentiality of further growth:

> Deck yourself out, if you can, in pride and dignity,
> array yourself in pomp and splendour;
> unleash the fury of your wrath,
> look upon the proud man and humble him;
> look upon every proud man and bring him low,
> throw down the wicked where they stand;
> hide them in the dust together,
> and shroud them in an unknown grave.
> Then I in my turn will acknowledge
> that your own right hand can save you.   (40: 9–14)

If, through the extremity of suffering, a state of humility is reached, it is possible then to find redemption. First it is necessary to lie down in the dust; later one can "stand up like a man".

Strength continues to be the source of the metaphors which follow. The wild ox, the horse, the hawk, the vulture, the whale and the crocodile are instanced for strength and skill beyond that of man. The New English Version boldly takes the "whale" and the "crocodile" as the translation of the words rendered "leviathan" and "behemoth", respectively, in the Authorized Version. Commentators have been in dispute as to whether these were mythical beasts or animals known in the Eastern Mediterranean region at that time. In the Soncino Version it is suggested that the leviathan stands for the crocodile and not the whale, whereas the behemoth, which literally is the plural form of the Hebrew word for beast or cattle, is taken, by virtue of its plurality, to imply immensity of size and to refer to the hippopotamus. Buxtorf is quoted as considering the description of the behemoth as being applicable to the elephant.[11]

[11] J. R. Dummelow (Ed.), *A Commentary on the Hebrew Bible* (London: Macmillan & Co., 1919).

The metaphor taken from the strength of these beasts is none the worse for the fact that human inventions and cunning have utilized some of their powers for man's own benefit. For those who hunt animals of legendary strength, the challenge is to mortal combat. The rules which men impose upon themselves in these trials of ultimate strength are as inexorable as those of the mediaeval tourney. Strength and skill are wagered, but there are the added hazards which come from blind fortune which favours one or other of the combatants. Van der Post took this theme as the basis of his novel *The Hunter and the Whale*.[12] The whale and the elephant stood as representation of supreme animal strength. Each is hunted for commercial purposes. In each case, however, the hunter personalizes his opponent and ties his destiny to his chosen quarry. In the novel, an unusually successful hunter of the whale, approaching the end of his vigour (but not his skill), has set himself the task of conquering a particular whale which had eluded all previous approaches. All the qualities of primitive power which could be opposed to man were embodied in this one specimen. Likewise, a hunter of the elephant, now in the climacteric of his strength, had determined to match himself against a particular elephant which was known by rumour rather than by the evidence of direct observation. In each case the quarry had been located, and at this point, by some quirk, the elephant hunter persuades the hunter of the whale to exchange objectives with him. The story ends tragically for them both; each had turned from the destiny which they separately had chosen. The destiny was the daemon which drives a man, and which is "that one talent which is death to hide".

Only a handful of men in any generation select themselves, or are selected, for this contest with primaeval forces which are symbolized here by the crocodile and the whale. Job stands as the representative of man when God taunted him with the question,

> Can you pull out the whale with a gaff
> or can you slip a noose round its tongue?
> Can you pass a cord through its nose
> or put a hook through its jaw?
>
> (41: 1–2)

---

[12] Laurens van der Post, *The Hunter and the Whale* (England: Penguin Books, 1970).

The reply could have been made that the time would come when man would accomplish these very feats but at great cost.

Taking the New English Bible rendering, it is the crocodile which is given descriptions applicable to power forever outside the bounds of the civilizing forces with which man identifies himself and endeavours to promulgate. This brute force is outside the purview of conscious, idealized man.

The attributes of the "crocodile" are that he is strong:

> What strength is in his loins!
> What power in the muscles of his belly!
>   (40:16)

aggressive:

> He is the chief of God's works,
> made to be a tyrant over his peers;
> for he takes the cattle of the hills for his prey
> and in his jaws he crunches all wild beasts.
>   (40:19–20)

concealed:

> There under the thorny lotus he lies,
> hidden in the reeds and the marsh;
> the lotus conceals him in its shadow,
> the poplars of the stream surround him.
>   (40:21–22)

unshackled:

> Can a man blind his eyes and take him
> or pierce his nose with the teeth of a trap?
> Can you fill his skin with harpoons
> or his head with fish-hooks?   (40:24, 41:7)

recoiling on any who attack:

> If ever you lift your hand against him,
> think of the struggle that awaits you, and let be.
> No, such a man is in desperate case,
> hurled headlong at the very sight of him.   (41:8–9)

ferocious:

> How fierce he is when he is roused!
> Who is there to stand up to him?

> Who has ever attacked him unscathed?
> Not a man under the wide heaven.
> > (41: 10–11)

but with a beauty in his strength:

> I will not pass over in silence his limbs,
> his prowess and the grace of his proportions.
> > (41: 12)

impenetrable in his outer defences:

> Who has ever undone his outer garment
> or penetrated his doublet of hide?
> . . .
> His back is row upon row of shields,
> enclosed in a wall of flints;
> one presses so close on the other
> that air cannot pass between them,
> each so firmly clamped to its neighbour
> that they hold and cannot spring apart.
> > (41: 13–17)

even more so is his centre secure:

> Close knit is his underbelly,
> no pressure will make it yield.
> His heart is firm as a rock,
> firm as the nether millstone.
> > (41: 23–24)

The attacks upon him by man are rendered feeble; weapons are of no avail:

> When he raises himself, strong men take fright,
> bewildered at the lashings of his tail.
> Sword or spear, dagger or javelin,
> if they touch him, they have no effect.
> Iron he counts as straw,
> and bronze as rotting wood.
> No arrow can pierce him,
> and for him sling-stones are turned into chaff;
> to him a club is a mere reed,
> and he laughs at the swish of the sabre.
> > (41: 25–29)

He is the dragon of legend:

> Firebrands shoot from his mouth,
> and sparks come streaming out;
> his nostrils pour forth smoke
> like a cauldron on a fire blown to full heat.
> His breath sets burning coals ablaze,
> and flames flash from his mouth.
>
> (41: 19–21)

He is the symbol of fearlessness and pride, the king of beasts:

> He has no equal on earth;
> for he is made quite without fear.
> He looks down on all creatures, even the highest;
> he is king over all proud beasts.   (41: 33–34)

We have quoted this final chapter of the speech out of the tempest almost in full, for in it are contained the representations of strength which Job needs to internalize. This strength had remained beyond Job's previous conscious contemplation.

Let us examine in detail what is implied in these descriptions of the "crocodile". Three important themes can be discerned: first, it is a metaphor for the being of God; secondly, for the dragon of mythology; and thirdly, it is a representation of man's unconscious. Jung deals with the second and third themes in Symbols of Transformation.[13]

The first theme is a view of God which is at variance with all Job's previous concepts. During the time that Job was calling God to account within the terms of moral determinacy, he had implicitly expected that any reply from God would of necessity be not only an answer to his charges, but would also be just, legalistic, rational, and predictable—in short, of the same nature as an answer which would have come from Job himself in his premorbid state of "perfection". But far from answering Job on Job's own premises, God replies obliquely (if not tangentially) by referring to the mysteries and the power of his creation, for which the crocodile stands as an example. Job had counted upon the mathematical equation of moral determinacy (e.g. a good life leads to good fortune), but the reply points to the unpredictable, ungovernable forces of nature which are outside moral laws. The moral order which Job had evoked as his

[13] C. G. Jung, *The Collected Works*, Vol. V (London: Routledge & Kegan Paul, 1956), pp. 374 ff.

defence is an anthropomorphic creation. The new concept, equated with the qualities of the crocodile, embraces aspects of nature beyond human ethics and ideology.

True though it is that Job earlier had accused God of being unjust, capricious, and unkind, he did so in order to bring God back to being the embodiment of the just, the reasonable, and the benevolent. There are many examples in Bible stories of God being appealed to, through prayer and conscious flattery, to represent the qualities which human beings desired in him. Job had used the opposite tactic, pointing out how God had deviated from man's ideal. Now, however, the strength and power of God's creative forces is being dissociated from the laws by which men govern their conscious lives.

The second theme to be discerned in the symbol of the crocodile is its relationship to the dragon of mythology (41: 19–21). This is the mythical beast which is depicted as being unconquerable; and yet, in every story in which it appears, whether it be terrorizing a city or holding a maiden in captivity, it is always conquered in the end by the hero, as a task in his initiation. If, as is here stated, the dragon is "king over all proud beasts" (41: 34), the man who conquers this symbol of pride is not only king over the king, but has conquered, in symbolic form, the area of pride within himself. It is a dangerous exploit to engage the dragon, and involves finding within oneself a power other than brute force—a more creative, ingenuous, uncalculating, semi-magical power in which new energies within the personality are released.

The ordeal has taken many forms. When Jacob wrestled "With God and with men" and prevailed, he asked for a blessing (Genesis 32: 25–31). The contradiction remains that, in wrestling with one's own pride, and finding humility in the defeat of that pride, there is a new pride in the victory. The reward comes in the experience that the man who humbles himself, saves himself (40: 9–14); and the one who saves himself, humbles himself. The humility, paradoxically, becomes the treasured possession.

In the third theme, it is possible to bring together the previous two. We can relate the attributes of the crocodile to the primitive aspects of man. It has already been noted that Job had on several occasions opened himself up to the experience of his own unconscious. Elihu had taken up the theme of the unconscious (33: 15–16) and had related the suffering involved in man's encounter with his inner self, to the price of his release from suffering. The crocodile, symbolizing the unconscious, has been invoked by Job (in so far as God's speech represents Job's thoughts) as the dynamic experience of his deepest unconscious mental processes. The unconscious is now seen as strong, aggressive, concealed, uncivilized, untamed, fierce, unscrutable, impenetrable, with a certain majestic beauty, and proud. Not to be in touch with it is a loss; actively to avoid a confrontation with it is a renunciation of an opportunity to develop further an integral part of the self.

Can any understand the spreadings of the Clouds
the noise of his Tabernacle

15

Also by watering he wearieth the thick cloud
He scattereth the bright cloud also it is turned about by his counsels

Of Behemoth he saith, He is the chief of the ways of God
Of Leviathan he saith, He is King over all the Children of Pride

Behold now Behemoth which I made with thee

W Blake invenit & sculpt

London Published as the Act directs March 8, 1825 by Will Blake N° 3 Fountain Court Strand

How precious are thy thoughts
unto me O God
how great is the sum of them

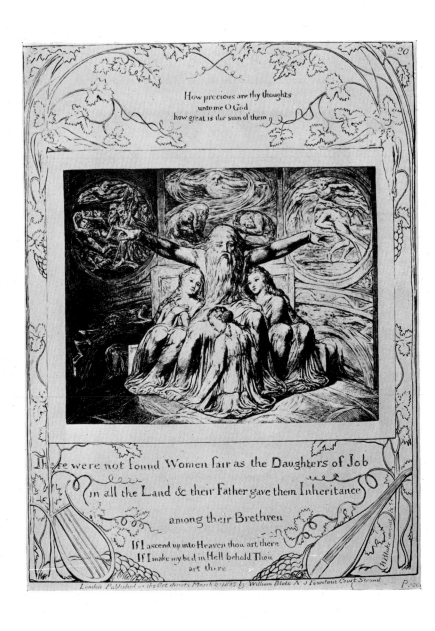

There were not found Women fair as the Daughters of Job

in all the Land & their Father gave them Inheritance

among their Brethren

If I ascend up into Heaven thou art there
If I make my bed in Hell behold Thou
art there

London Published as the Act directs March 8: 1825 by William Blake N 3 Fountain Court Strand.

CHAPTER 9

The Inner Consummation

AT this point we wish to introduce a new thought about the transformation of Job. The final Job is neither the old Job restored to health, nor a new Job with qualities different from the old one. It is, instead, a consummation of qualities previously outlined but not fully developed. The turbulence of the tempest out of which God spoke had had its reflection within Job, and he was able to turn around some of his own sayings and convert them from vituperation to insight. When Elihu advanced the thought that a mediator, an interpreter, could help Job find the price of his release, the phrase used was "if an angel, one of thousands, stands by him" (33: 23). In rabbinical legends, the angels which stand by a man at the time of judgement are his good deeds and bad deeds (and, for that matter, his good thoughts and his bad thoughts). One good deed amongst a thousand human failings might well be the price of a man's release. One normal strand in the pattern of mental disorder may carry a man back to sanity. Job had used the example of the "one in a thousand" (9: 3) at an earlier stage without being able to give it a reassuring meaning. Here, the New English Version attributes the "one in a thousand" to God's answer to the question of man:

> "If a man chooses to argue with him,
> God will not answer one question in a thousand",

but adds, as a footnote, the reverse interpretation, viz.

> "If God is pleased to argue with him, man
> cannot answer one question in a thousand".

The Soncino Version quotes one commentator:

> "If the righteous desired to dispute with the Omnipresent concerning the out-
> rage of witholding His reward, he could not even give him one answer out
> of His thousand questions".   (Metsudah David)

It is only one step, but a significant one, from being unable to answer
one question in a thousand to gaining the capacity to be right that once
in a thousand. To be right once in a thousand is sufficient to restore the
inner confidence in his salvation:

> But in my heart I know that my vindicator lives
> and that he will rise last to speak in court;
> and I shall discern my witness standing at my side
> and see my defending counsel, even God himself,
> whom I shall see with my own eyes,
> I myself and no other.   (19: 25–27)

These words were prophetic. Job was finally able to say:

> I knew of thee then only by report,
> but now I see thee with my own eyes.
>   (42: 5)

But God did not appear within the habitual trappings of a heavenly
court modelled on an earthly counterpart. Job's vision is of a God of
whom there was no pre-existing image. Job's insight was his own
("... God himself, whom I shall see with my own eyes, I myself and no
other"). Neither the comforters nor Elihu give an indication that they
had heard or had seen God in his appearance out of the tempest. God is
thus Job's inner experience, a "revelation", which was personal to him.

This is the penultimate crisis. Job's inner experience of God is in direct
opposition to his lifelong conscious conception. The collision between
Job's contention of the unjustness of his trials and his concept of a good
and reasonable God had aggravated his suffering; and, at the height of his
sufferings, a perfect Job was the victim of an imperfect God. The premorbid, perfect Job had been a human reproduction of an equally perfect
God. During the illness, his capacity to find imperfections in God heralded
his subsequent discovery of his own human imperfections. The new God
contained all the powers perceivable in nature. The new God was an
integration of the whole of nature. This new God would not need a

Satan to point out the imperfection in God's creatures, because he would include all the qualities which Job was able to conceive in the universe. In a less explicit way, Job would be able to extend his previous conscious view of his own self and to acknowledge that his previous perfect and upright image must have concealed imperfections. We have referred to him as being "integrated", but his integrity was previously maintained only by ignoring the existence of qualities which were considered bad.

In the time scale of the narrative, some considerable duration must be allotted to the mental processes involved in Job's projection and reintrojection of qualities in God. This could have already been taking place in the unspoken associations to his own and his comforters' speeches. Formulation needs time. Unconscious turmoil is non-verbal. The conflict between old ideas and the emerging new ones is the generator of anxieties that are almost too great to bear. New ideas are understandably to be feared. The old ones had the safety of familiarity; the new ones could be found wanting; and the substitution of new for old is a disloyalty to one's inheritance.

If justice should stand for the highest level of man's perfection, the sacrifice of perfection would make it necessary to relinquish the hope of receiving justice. Job had demanded justice, and he had found that justice was too threatening a concept, since all who aim at perfection, and fail, must suffer judgement of their imperfection. The escape from this dilemma was the acceptance of indeterminism, which includes recognition of the irrational in man, the unpredictable in nature, and unfairness in the relationships of man and God.

Job had gradually been building up a foundation of religious thought based upon his own observations of animate and inanimate nature, and he had found his observations to be inconsistent with traditional beliefs. At the moment when Job hears and sees God, he has to give up his self-concept of perfection. His problem now is to find a new definition of himself which will be in harmony with his vision of the profusion and variegation in nature.

The revelation of God gives Job a final victory over his comforters' challenges, at the expense of his own pride. God's speech ends with the idea of pride: the last line is, "he is king over all proud beasts". Job's reply and final comment is essentially concerned with humility. Job's new-found humility, brief though it may prove to be, has the incalculable importance that within it was found the new self-concept of Job:

> I know that thou canst do all things
> and that no purpose is beyond thee.
> But I have spoken of great things which I have not understood,
> things too wonderful for me to know.
> I knew of thee then only by report,
> but now I see thee with my own eyes.
> Therefore I melt away;
> I repent in dust and ashes.   (42: 2–6)

Never before had Job been able to admit his presumption. The feeling of shame now gives way to a feeling of awe. He acknowledges that man can no longer hope to have control over God, or even over his own fate. In one single verse, Job wipes out the contractual relationship which his religious predecessors had established in the Covenants between God and man and man and God.[1]

> I know that thou canst do all things
> and that no purpose is beyond thee.
> (42: 2)

The implementation by God of such Covenants could always be demanded by man, but Job abrogates this power. He renounces his claim to equality in law, power, and knowledge:

> But I have spoken of great things which I have not understood,
> things too wonderful for me to know.   (42: 3)

While recognizing the limitations of his former understanding, he welcomes the new insight which he has gained:

> I knew of thee then only by report,
> but now I see thee with my own eyes.
> (42: 5)

Lastly, he recognizes the new humility which is a consciousness of his human condition:

> Therefore I melt away;
> I repent in dust and ashes.
> (42: 6)

---

[1] Noah (Genesis 10: 9–17), Abraham (Genesis 17: 1–11).

The Soncino publication points out that the literal translation for the Hebrew word for "melt away" is "I abhor". Job does not say "I abhor *myself*"; he is acknowledging his *abhoring* in an intransitive sense. Job is now able to recognize the hatred in himself (his bad side); at the same time, he recognizes his shame ("I repent"). This makes it possible for him to look upon his hate as being good. It is bad to hate, but it is good to be able to acknowledge the hatred, and to repent.

There is a charming example of this mental manoeuvre in the analysis of a phobia in a five-year-old boy conducted by the boy's father under the guidance and instruction of Freud. The boy revealed to his father that he wished that his younger sister was not alive. In the conversation recorded by the father, for transmission to Freud, there is the following sequence:

Father: "A good boy doesn't wish that sort of thing."
Hans: "But he may THINK it."
Father: "But that isn't good."
Hans: "If he thinks it, it IS good all the same, because you can write it to the Professor."[2]

In Job's case he repents wholeheartedly, and no doubt derives positive pleasure from the goodness of his repentance. As with little Hans, it was turned to good use!

But Job, however, goes further than repentance in his state of abhorring. The word abhor has a secondary meaning, "to shrink back in dread and terror". This implies the feeling of awe to which reference has already been made. Shame, hate, repentance, and, finally, awe—these are feelings to which the former Job would never have admitted. He has acknowledged the complexity of the self which encompasses good and bad, and this was possible only after he had been able to apprehend a God who himself comprehends all possibilities: good and bad, known and unknown, finite and infinite. No longer can he call himself "perfect". Above all else, we can discern the humanization of Job.

"In dust and ashes" is rendered in the Soncino Version as "*seeing* I am dust and ashes", i.e. human, mortal. The return to dust and ashes is the completion of the cycle of life and refers to death. The phrase is quoted in the religious service for the dead in which it is also said that "for there is not a righteous man on earth who doeth good and sinneth not". In

[2] Sigmund Freud, *Standard Edition*, Vol. X (London: Hogarth Press, 1955), p. 72.

order to rid himself of the perfection of his righteousness Job had to bury his former self. We can now look upon what follows as a rebirth. The culmination of the therapeutic process is the beginning of a new life.

We shall need to define or describe the identity of the reborn Job. The word *tam* is still applicable, not in its original meaning of "perfect", but *tam* in its meaning of completeness, wholeness—the integration of good and bad.

In this short speech—Job shows that he has incorporated those parts which he had denied—the shame, the awe, the humanity. Job began with the *tam* of perfection; he ends with the *tam* of integration. He has accomplished the price of his release from his perfection.

No sooner had Job become aware of his inner imperfection, than he once again becomes interpreter, intermediary, and mediator with God on behalf of the comforters.

The Epilogue, which rounds off the story, structurally resembles the Prologue, in that it is written in prose. Superficially, it might appear that Job ends as he began, with his fortunes restored and with a new family to replace the old. Our contention is, however, that there would be an inevitable difference between the old Job and the new. In the terms of the Bible narrative, the circumstances of his recovery are themselves an indication that changes have taken place in Job.

The first indication is God's anger towards the comforters. During his illness, Job had been angry with them, and they with him, and this resulted in an impasse. The anger towards them now becomes the anger of God and not that of Job. This anger can be used constructively to lift them up again. But even more so is Job lifted up in his re-established relationship with God.

> When the LORD had finished speaking to Job, he said to Eliphaz the Temanite, "I am angry with you and your friends, because you have not spoken as you ought about me, as my servant Job has done. So now take seven bulls and seven rams, go to my servant Job, and offer a whole-offering for yourselves, and he will intercede for you; I will surely show him favour by not being harsh with you because you have not spoken as you ought about me, as he has done."
> (42: 7-8)

The comforters are made to resume the inferior position towards Job which they had occupied before Job had sustained his losses. It is the comforters' turn to seek help from Job; Job has again acquired a special position with God. God chooses Job as the intercessor for the comforters, and only through the person of Job would God pardon them. This was evidence of Job's renewal of potency in the priestly qualities of his role as patriarch. Job's former superior position *vis-à-vis* the comforters, which had temporarily been reversed, is now renewed. The harmonious relationship which Job had enjoyed with God, which was dissipated during the time of his illness, has been restored. It was necessary for Job to destroy his special relationship with God in order to achieve his cure, and it became necessary for him to create a new relationship in order to fulfill the personality that emerged from the suffering. The cycle is not complete until Job has interceded for his friends. First of all the comforters were required to make their offering through Job in order to avoid God's disfavour towards them. In this way they were forced to pay tribute to Job's superior insight at this moment.

In the world of psychotherapy, it is not infrequent for the recovered patient to become the therapist to others; and Job's first task after his illness, which was also his first honour and privilege, was to receive homage from the comforters and be the agent of their redemption.

The consequential reward to Job for his first practical act was that God would not be harsh to his friends and that they would not have to suffer as Job had just done. It was only when Job had completed his task that God made a direct repayment to him:

> Then Eliphaz the Temanite and Bildad the Shuhite and Zophar the Naamathite went and carried out the LORD's command, and the LORD showed favour to Job *when* he had interceded for his friends. So the LORD restored Job's fortunes and doubled all his possessions [*our italics*].   (42: 9–10)

After God had shown favour to Job once more, it became possible for his relatives and friends, who had deserted him in his troubles, to make amends:

> Then all Job's brothers and sisters and his former acquaintance came and feasted with him in his home, and they consoled and comforted him for all the misfortunes which the LORD had brought on him; and each of them gave him a sheep and a gold ring.   (42: 11)

It is significant that they now reappear when once again Job takes up his position as head of his family. The feast which they share with Job at his home is a celebration of his return to good health and good fortune, and the presents which they offer to him are symbolic of their recognition of his patriarchal status.

> Furthermore, the LORD blessed the end of Job's life more than the beginning; and he had fourteen thousand head of small cattle and six thousand camels, a thousand yoke of oxen and as many she-asses. He had seven sons and three daughters;   (42: 12–13)

Job's material possessions are returned in double measure. His sons and daughters are in number as before, but to his daughters Job gives names and inheritance:

> and he named his eldest daughter Jemimah, the second Keziah, and the third Kerenhappuch. There were no women in all the world so beautiful as Job's daughters; and their father gave them an inheritance with their brothers.
> (42: 14–15)

In the ancient Hebraic laws no inheritance was provided for the daughters; only the sons enjoyed such recognition from their fathers. Here, by naming his daughters and giving them an inheritance, Job makes recognition of the equal claim of the female to the birthright which, in the Biblical sense, is a spiritual blessing as well as a material possession. (The names of the sons are not given in the Bible text, so that we may take this emphasis on the daughters as significant.) Job, as the male head of the family, the patriarch—its father and priest—defied tradition by granting recognition of feminine rights. There is a hint here of a new importance to Job of the father–daughter relationship. This relationship is a somewhat neglected feature in the discussion of a number of Shakespearian characters and we shall draw attention to it in our conclusions.

And so the Book of Job ends:

> Thereafter Job lived another hundred and forty years, he saw his sons and his grandsons to four generations, and died at a very great age.   (42: 16–17)

Job's virility and his monumental strength are returned to him in great measure. As Elihu indicated, concerning the restoration of the man who can recognize the badness within himself, "then that man will grow sturdier than he was in youth" (33: 25).

The drama ends when Job's losses are restored, but his life goes on until, in the words of the Authorized Version, he ". . . died, being old and full of days." The days were full of life. Likewise our theme of an illness and its cure comes to an end, but other thoughts continue.

We have postulated earlier that the essential quality in Job's cure was to release himself from obsessional insistence on exact measure in relationships between man and man, and between man and God. This release involves the ability to settle for less than is one's due. At the same time it requires the preparedness to accept graciously more than is one's due. The bonus which comes without one necessarily having deserved it may seem to be a burden to some people. It is a fairly general attitude to treat unexpected gifts as if they had to be paid for in due course. It is even said of fine weather, "We shall have to pay for this later." But it is just as much a sign of maturity to accept gifts with a good grace as to be able to carry the hurt of unexpected losses.

It is part of the human condition to undergo, in different degrees, some of the suffering of Job. Our interpretation is not intended to be a definitive account of all illness, of all suffering, or of all the vicissitudes and vagaries of fortune which human beings undergo. It would not be possible in these days to conclude as Moses Maimonides did:

> If you pay to my words the attention which this treatise demands, and examine all that is said in the Book of Job, all will be clear to you, and you will find that I have grasped and taken hold of the whole subject; nothing has been left unnoticed, except such portions as are only introduced because of the context and the whole plan of the allegory. I have explained this method several times in the course of this treatise.[3]

Presumptuous though this claim may have seemed, Maimonides had in fact touched upon many themes not dealt with in other writings on the Book of Job. He distinguishes the meanings of the word "rule" (or "laws"), as applied to God, from the meaning that we use "when we rule over other beings". In the same manner, he stated "there is a difference between the rules which apply to natural forces and the moral rules which apply to our conduct." The difference is clearly between scientific laws, moral laws, and the laws of government.

Maimonides commented: "it is remarkable . . . that wisdom is not ascribed to Job. The text does not say he was an intelligent, wise, or clever man; but virtue and uprightness, especially in actions, are ascribed to him." It is possible for us to be carried away by the richness of Job's

[3] Moses Maimonides, *op. cit.*, p. 303.

imagery, and thereby to be lost in admiration of his character, but it would not be too much to say that Job was a tiresome old man (and perhaps lovable in spite of it). At this point we wish to introduce a comparison, already hinted at, between Job and some Shakesperian characters. This comparison is with three tiresome old men—Polonius, King Lear, and Prospero. All three were portrayed in juxtaposition with their daughters. Polonius, who is best remembered for his moment of sincerity when addressing his son ("This above all; to thine own self be true"), was anything but sincere in his dealings with Ophelia. His advice to her with regard to Hamlet was governed by his wish to serve the queen and the usurping king. Ophelia's death was due as much to his compromising schemes as to anything else. He lost a daughter to his petty ambition. King Lear was betrayed by two of his daughters and he himself betrayed the daughter whom he loved the most. His hidden love, and hers, stood between them and the sincerity of their communication. But the rebellion of the older daughters was of Lear's own making. The inheritance which he gave them in his own lifetime was hedged with implied conditions. Their enjoyment of it was subject to Lear's prior claim to them and to the possessions which he had handed over. In just such a manner Job had sacrificed to God to make good the wantonness of the expenditure of his children.

Prospero succeeded where the others failed. He too lost his daughter, but he lost her to marriage, although he managed to prolong the process of his daughter's liberation. It is interesting that the island exile, where Prospero developed his magical powers, began with a tempest and ended with a tempest. As with Job, the "Tempest" was reflected by conflicting elements within. The storm gathered, then broke, and in the ensuing calm a new balance was achieved.

When the time came for Prospero to enlighten his daughter as to her origin, he took off his magical cloak and became simply her father. When they left the island he cast away his magical cloak forever. The father-daughter relationship was consummated by their freedom to separate from one another and by Prospero's abrogation of his omnipotence.

Prospero's life had a cycle somewhat comparable with that of Job. Prospero, like Job, was a great man. He was stripped of his ducal possessions, but escaped with life and his only daughter. In the enclosed world of the island he became exalted, used magical powers to challenge and control the whole of nature; but the consummation was to reconcile himself with the limited yet responsible duties of the ordinary great man! Job's cycle of life has already been considered by us in many dimensions. Our first theme utilized the model of health/illness/cure. We elaborated this by studying the premorbid qualities of personality which had inevitably led to the illness. We also tried to indicate the creative and positive qualities of the experiences which we have called symptoms. We do not wish to minimize the severity of Job's sufferings, nor do we wish to imply that mental illness is intrinsically a beneficial experience. Yet there are instances where it is through a mental disorder that an individual is able to seek and find the understanding which takes him to higher developments of personality. Sometimes it is the therapist (Elihu's inter-mediary) who takes the sufferer to the new levels. There are others who struggle alone through the depths of despair to the insights which can come only from a turmoil which brings unconscious mental processes into one's awareness.

Ellenberger discusses the emergence of revolutionary psychological theory in the work of Fechner, Jung, and Freud as the result of what he calls a creative illness. Each of these innovators underwent periods of mental disturbance at the time of their most intensive productivity.

> A creative illness succeeds a period of intense preoccupation with an idea and search for a certain truth. It is a polymorphous condition that can take the shape of depression, neurosis, psychosomatic ailments, or even psychosis. Whatever the symptoms, they are felt as painful, if not agonizing, by the subject, with alternating periods of alleviation and worsening. Throughout the illness the subject never loses the thread of his dominating preoccupation. It is often compatible with normal, professional activity and family life. But even if he keeps to his social activities, he is almost entirely absorbed with himself. He suffers from feelings of utter isolation, even when he has a mentor who guides him through the ordeal (like the shaman apprentice with his master). The termina-tion is often rapid and marked by a phase of exhilaration. The subject emerges from his ordeal with a permanent transformation in his personality and the conviction that he has discovered a great truth or a new spiritual world.[4]

Without too much support from the text we have tried to infer that, at the end of the cycle of illness, Job has used the creative imagery of his own words, the speech of Elihu, and the revelation from the tempest, to

[4] H. F. Ellenberger, *The Discovery of the Unconscious* (London: Allen Lane, The Penguin Press, 1970), pp. 447–448.

find a more serene and balanced personality, and eventually he could consent to his own mortality.

In these considerations we have taken the jump from the cycle of health/illness/cure to the cycle of obsessional preoccupation/depression/creative insight. Another variant of this cycle would be perfectionism/disintegration/integration.

The same sequential pattern can also be described in terms which recognize the contribution of the surrounding culture to personality changes in an individual. This contribution is reciprocal: there are individuals who are changed by the culture and there are those who are the agents of cultural change. These latter agents are not like the therapists of individual sufferers. They relate themselves to the total community in which they live. They are the revolutionaries or, in Biblical times, the prophets. For a short period in his life Job was a prophet. The cycle here was patriarch/prophet/patriarch.

The prophet makes his appearance during the transitional stages in civilizations, and such a stage occurred in European history at the beginning of the nineteenth century when religious and political traditionalism was challenged by new scientific discoveries. There was a special case later in the century when some of the Jewish ghettoes opened themselves to the influence of the new learning. There was opposition between universalism and nationalism, religion and science, and between spiritual and material values. Ahad Ha'am was a writer who tried to preserve the spiritual quality that was in danger of being lost in the exit from the ghetto. He challenged some of the features of narrow nationalism, but was equally critical of the message which some intellectuals were finding in the teachings of Nietzsche. In one of his essays, Ahad Ha'am discusses the qualities of the prophet which distinguishes him from the rest of mankind.

First, the prophet is a man of truth. He sees life as it is, undistorted by subjective feelings, and tells what he sees unaffected by irrelevant considerations. He tells the truth, not because he is convinced that such is his duty, but because truth telling is a characteristic of which he cannot rid himself even if he would.

Secondly, the prophet is an extremist. He can consent to no compromise, and can never cease thundering his passionate denunciation, even if the whole universe is against him.

The third characteristic is a resultant of the other two, and is the supremacy of absolute righteousness in the prophet's every word and action. As an extremist, he cannot subordinate righteousness any more than he can subordinate truth.

The prophet, therefore, is in the difficult position that, on the one hand, he cannot altogether reform the world according to his desire; on the other hand, he cannot deceive himself and shut his eyes to its defects. Hence, it is impossible for him ever to be at peace with the actual life in which his days are spent.[5]

There is a corollary from Ahad Ha'am's formulations of the prophet. The prophet can never be a family man. As a patriarch, Job was priest and father of a family, as well as a man of affairs. He was a prophet in the interval when he had lost his family and his possessions. His new life, at the conclusion when his possessions were doubly restored, may have involved some compromise.

Lionel Trilling quotes Rousseau on Molière's *Le Misanthrope*, stating that it represented "a false good, more dangerous than actual evil" and making *"wisdom consist in a certain mean between vice and virtue"*.[6] The view that Job's final position included such a compromise is moderated somewhat by Job's access to shame and awe.

The final dimension is the general philosophical position in which man has to choose between the assumption that the universe is understandable and the assumption that there will always be phenomena beyond comprehension. The first assumption is the act of faith behind all science. We seek to understand natural phenomena and we therefore are required to believe in the law of causality, i.e. the same causes always have the same effects. By studying effects we infer causes; and any effect for which no cause is discoverable still has its cause—which will be discovered at some time in the future. The alternative viewpoint is that, no matter how much has been discovered and which will be discovered in the future, some aspects of the universe will always remain beyond human comprehension.

These opposite principles are represented in human thinking by the ideas of determinism and indeterminism. The principle of determinism

[5] Ahad Ha'am, *Selected Essays*, transl. Leon Simon (Philadelphia: The Jewish Publication Society of America, 1912), pp. 311–313.

[6] Lionel Trilling, *op. cit.*, pp. 17–18 *(our italics)*.

was convincingly applied to some very simple relationships which were expressed as laws of science; and these are the foundations of physics and chemistry. These principles were transferred to living as well as inorganic matter, and the science of biology was created. More recently there have been extensions of the principle to the study of human relationships and to the inner processes of the human mind. The latter is expressed as psychic determinism. Surprisingly, the idea of moral determinacy is older than physical and psychic determinism. In all these worlds of thought there has been a corresponding and co-existing principle of indeterminacy which, for some reason, has seemed less attractive. Many people seem to prefer to believe that the concept of chance is somehow unscientific, and that the idea of chance would disappear if we were able to correlate all the operating factors. The confusion is between two meanings of the word "law", the confusion which Maimonides pointed out as existing between the laws which human beings make, and which have to be obeyed, as against the laws of nature which are merely the regularities which have been observed.

There is a certain amount of emotion attached to the consideration of indeterminism.[7] The issue is similar to that of ambivalence, which is the simultaneous existence of love and hate. The same considerations are also attached to the topic of death. The declared aim of the remedial services, which human beings have created, is to cure or to prevent disease and, it is implied, to prevent death. But illness and death are facts of life. Some illnesses are traced to causes which are preventable, and some pathological processes are curable. There are diseases which formerly were incurable which now come under cure. But there are illnesses which remain incurable and death does not always wait extreme old age. Although we know why some diseases and misfortunes occur, and why in the civilized lives that we live we face hazards of accident, as well as of ill fortune, we do not know which particular person will suffer a calamity in which there is a statistically precise, predictable incidence.

Some of these ideas have been enclosed in the concept of destiny which helps people to accommodate to the events which we cannot determine. The awe, which is Job's tribute to destiny, is the final acknowledgement of the mortality of man.

[7] J. H. Kahn, "Beyond the determinacy principle", *Applied Social Studies*, **1** (1969), pp. 73–80.

Bibliography

THE BIBLE

Wycliffite Version of the Bible, Wycliffite, Hereford, Purvey, 1381/1388, edited by Waltar W. Skeat, Oxford University Press, 1880.
Authorized Version of the Bible, 1611.
Revised Version of the Bible, 1885.
Soncino Books of the Bible: *Job*, Soncino Press, Eng., 1946, Eng. trans. by The Jewish Publication Society of America.
The Septuagint Bible, trans. Charles Thomson, Rev., C. A. Muses, Colorado, The Falcon's Wing Press, 1954.
The New English Bible, Oxford University Press and Cambridge University Press, 1970.

BIBLE COMMENTARIES

COBBIN, Ingram, Rev., *The Condensed Commentary and Family Exposition of the Holy Bible*, Thomas Ward & Co., London, 1839.
DUMMELOW, J. R., Rev. (Ed.), *A Commentary on the Holy Bible*, Macmillan & Co., London, 1919.
Jewish Encyclopedia, Vol. II, Funk & Wagnall's, New York, 1902.
MAIMONIDES, Moses (1168), *The Guide for the Perplexed*, trans. M. Friedlander, George Routledge & Sons, London, 1947.

LITERARY, PHILOSOPHICAL AND HISTORICAL

AHAD HA'AM, *Selected Essays*, trans. Leon Simon, The Jewish Publication Society of America, Philadelphia, 1912.
BLAKE, William, *An Illustrated Catalogue of Works in the Fitzwilliam Museum Cambridge*, Ed. Bindman, D., Syndics of the Fitzwilliam Museum, Cambridge.

BLAKE, William, *Illustrations of the Book of Job*, reproduced and reduced facsimile from impressions in the British Museum, Gowans & Graye, 1927.

BLAKE, William, *Complete Writings*, Oxford University Press, 1966.

BURTON, Robert (1621), *Anatomy of Melancholy*.

CAMPBELL, Joseph, *The Hero with a Thousand Faces*, 2nd ed., Princeton University Press, New Jersey, 1968.

DENNIS, Nigel, *Cards of Identity*, William Clowes & Sons, London, 1955.

FROUDE, J. A., *Short Studies on Great Subjects*, J. M. Dent & Sons, London, 1906.

GOLLANCZ, Victor, *From Darkness to Light*, Gollancz, London, 1956.

HUXLEY, Aldous, *Ends and Means*, Chatto & Windus, London, 1938.

HUXLEY, Julian, *Essays of a Biologist*, Chatto & Windus, London, 1923.

KALLEN, Horace M., *The Book of Job as a Greek Tragedy*, Hill & Wang, New York, 1918.

MACLEISH, Archibald, *J.B.*, Houghton Mifflin Company, Boston, 1956.

MANN, Thomas, *The Magic Mountain*, Martin Secker Ltd., London, 1927.

MILTON, John, *Samson Agonistes*.

SHAKESPEARE, William, *Hamlet, King Lear, The Tempest, The Sonnets*.

TRILLING, Lionel, *Sincerity and Authenticity*, Oxford University Press, London, 1972.

VAN DER POST, Laurens, *The Hunter and the Whale*, Penguin Books, England, 1970.

WHITE, Patrick, *Voss*, Eyre & Spottiswoode, 1957.

MEDICAL, PSYCHIATRIC AND PSYCHOLOGICAL

BATESON, G., JACKSON, D. D., HALEY, J., *et al.*, "Toward a theory of schizophrenia", *Behav. Sci.* **1** (1956), pp. 251–264.

BENNETT, Sir Risdon, *The Diseases of the Bible*, Horace Hart, Oxford, 1887.

BLANK, Leonard, *et al.* (Ed.), *Confrontation—Encounters in Self and Interpersonal Awareness*, The Macmillan Company, New York, 1971.

BOWLBY, John, *Attachment and Loss, Vol. II, Separation, Anxiety and Anger*. Hogarth Press, London, 1973.

BOYERS, Robert, and ORRILL, Robert (Ed.), *Laing and Anti-Psychiatry*, Penguin Education, London, 1972.

BRIM, Charles, "Job's illness—pellagra", *Archives of Dermatology and Syphilology*, **46** (2), (Feb. 1942), pp. 371–376.

BROWN, M. Webster, "Was Job a leper?", *Medical Journal and Record*, (July 1933), pp. 32–33.

CAPLAN, G., *Concepts of Mental Health Consultation*, Children's Bureau, U.S. Dept. of H.E.W., 1959.

COLEMAN, Jules, "Social factors influencing the development and containment of psychiatric symptoms", in J. J. Scheff, *Mental Illness and Social Processes*, Harper & Row, New York, 1947.

ELLENBERGER, H. F., *The Discovery of the Unconscious*, Allen Lane, The Penguin Press, London, 1970.

ERIKSON, Erik H., *Childhood and Society*, W. W. Norton & Co., New York, 1950.

FENICHEL, Otto, *The Psychoanalytic Theory of Neurosis*, W. W. Norton & Co., New York, 1945.

FORTES, Meyer, *Oedipus and Job in West African Religion*, Cambridge University Press, 1959.

FREUD, Sigmund, *Collected Papers, Vol. II*, Hogarth Press, London, 1948 (*The Psychogenesis of a Case of Homosexuality in a Woman*, 1920).

FREUD, Sigmund, *Collected Papers, Vol. III*, Ed. Ernest Jones, Hogarth Press, London, 1948.

FREUD, Sigmund, *Collected Papers, Vol. IV*, Ed. Ernest Jones, Hogarth Press, London, 1948.

FREUD, Sigmund, *Standard Edition, Vol. X*, London, Hogarth Press, 1955.

FROMM, Erich, *You shall be as Gods*, Jonathan Cape, London, 1967.

GLOVER, Edward, *Psycho-Analysis*, Staples Press, London, 1949.

GREENSON, Ralph R., *The Technique and Practice of Psycho-Analysis*, Vol. I, The Hogarth Press, 1967.

GUY, William, "Psychosomatic dermatology *circa* 400 B.C.", *Archives of Dermatology and Syphilology*, **71** (3), (March 1955), pp. 354–356.

HALLIDAY, James, *Psychosocial Medicine*, Heinemann, London, 1948.

HALLIDAY, James, "Psychosomatic medicine and the rheumatism problem", *The Practitioner*, **152** (Jan. 1944), pp. 6–15.

Henderson & Guillespie's Textbook of Psychiatry, rev. by Ivor Batchelor, 10th Ed., Oxford University Press, London, 1969.

HENRY, Jules, *Pathways to Madness*, Jonathan Cape, London, 1972.

HOLBROOK, David, *Human Hope and the Death Instinct*, Pergamon Press, Oxford, 1971.

JACOBI, Jolande, *The Psychology of C. G. Jung*, Routledge & Kegan Paul, London, 1942.

JONES, Ernest, *Sigmund Freud: Life and Work*, Vol. I, Hogarth Press, London, 1953.

JUNG, Carl, *Answer to Job*, trans. R. F. C. Hull, Hodder & Stoughton, London, 1964.

JUNG, C. G., *The Collected Works, Vol. V: Symbols of Transformation*, Routledge & Kegan Paul, London, 1959.

KAFKA, J. S., "Ambiguity for Individuation", *Arch. Gen. Psychiat.* **25** (Sept. 1971)

KAHN, J. H., "Beyond the determinacy principle", *Applied Social Studies*, **1** (1969).

KAHN, J. H., *Human Growth and Development of Personality*, 2nd Ed., Pergamon Press, Oxford, 1971.

KLEIN, D. C. and LINDEMANN, E., "Preventive intervention in individual and family crisis situations", in Gerald Caplan (Ed.), *Prevention of Mental Disorders in Children*, pp. 283–306, Tavistock Publications Ltd., London, 1961.

KLEIN, Melanie, *Our Adult World and Other Essays*, Heinemann, London, 1963.

LAING, R. D. *The Divided Self*, Tavistock Publications, London, 1960.

LAING, R. D., *The Self and Others*, Tavistock Publications, London, 1961.

LEWIS, Aubrey, "Psychological medicine", in F. W. Price (Ed.), *A Textbook of the Practice of Medicine*, Oxford University Press, London, 1947.

LIBRARIAN, Army Medical Library, "Morbus Jobi", *The Urologic and Cutaneous Review*, **40** (1936), pp. 296–299.

LINDEMANN, E., "Symptomatology and management of acute grief", *Am. J. Psychiat.* **101** (1944), pp. 1D.

MILNER, Marion, "The sense in non-sense—Freud and Blake's Job", *Freud, Jung and Adler; Their Relevance to the Teacher's Life and Work*, reprinted from *The New Era*, **1** (Jan. 1956).

NAGERA, Dr. Humberto, *et al.*, *Basic Psychoanalytical Concepts on the Libido Theory*, Ruskin House, London, 1969.

PARKES, C. Murray, "Attachment and autonomy at the end of life", in Gosling, R. (Ed.), *Support, Innovation and Autonomy*, Tavistock Publications, London, 1973.

RENDLE-SHORT, A., *The Bible and Modern Medicine*, Paternoster Press, London, 1953.

ROBINSON, David, *Patients, Practitioners and Medical Care—Aspects of Medical Sociology*, William Heinemann Medical Books Ltd., London, 1973.

SATIR, Virginia, *Conjoint Family Therapy*, rev. ed., Science and Behavior Books, Calif., 1967.

SCHEFF, Thomas J., *Mental Illness and Social Process*, Harper & Row, London, 1967.

SHANDS, Harley C., "The war with words", in J. Masserman (Ed.), *Communication and Community*, Grune & Stratton, New York, 1965.

SLUZKI and VERON, "The double bind as a universal pathogenic situation", *Family Process*, **10** (1971), as abstracted by Elizabeth Groff, *Digest of Neurology and Psychiatry*, **39** (Dec. 1971).

STEKEL, Wilhelm, *Compulsion and Doubt*, trans. Emil A. Gutheil, Liveright Publishing Corp., New York, 1949.

STOLLER, F. H., "A stage for trust", in A. Burton (Ed.), *Encounter: The Theory and Practice of Encounter Groups*, Jossey-Bass, San Francisco, 1969.

STORR, A., *The Integrity of Personality*, Penguin Books, Middlesex, 1965.

SZASZ, T. S., *The Manufacture of Madness*, Routledge & Kegan Paul, London, 1971.

SZASZ, T. S., "The myth of mental illness", in T. Scheff, (Ed.), *Mental Illness and Social Processes*, Harper & Row, New York, 1967.

THOMPSON, S. and KAHN, J., *The Group Process as a Helping Technique*, Pergamon Press, Oxford, 1970.

WHITAKER, D. S., and LIEBERMAN, M. A., *Psychotherapy through the Group Process*, Tavistock Publications, London, 1965.

WINNICOTT, D. W., "The family affected by depressive illness in one or both parents", 1958, in *The Family and Individual Development*, Tavistock Publications, London, 1965.

Index